B WILKINSON.

ANOTHER DOOR OPENS

Best Wishes
Margaret Wynne
Jack Wynne

HUMAN HORIZONS SERIES

ANOTHER DOOR OPENS

by

Margaret and Jack Wymer

A CONDOR BOOK
SOUVENIR PRESS (E & A) LTD

First published 1980 by Souvenir Press (Educational & Academic) Ltd,
43 Great Russell Street, London WC1B 3PA
and simultaneously in Canada

ISBN 0 285 64910 8 casebound
ISBN 0 285 64911 6 paperback

Printed in Great Britain by
Clarke, Doble & Brendon Ltd,
Plymouth and London

DEDICATED
TO THE INSPIRATION
AND THE MEMORY
OF
ELIZABETH BARNES

ACKNOWLEDGING
THE KIND INTEREST AND ASSISTANCE
OF
MEMBERS OF THE
NORWICH WRITERS' CIRCLE

REMEMBERING
MY DEAR FATHER
AND SHEILA

Contents

Why Write a Book?

We have altered our attitudes to this book over the period of writing it. At first we wanted, rightly or wrongly, to show other disabled people what could be achieved, given the correct set of circumstances. Then we thought that perhaps those in authority might be inspired to provide the necessary conditions for independence for other disabled. Certainly in our case, it was having one such personality who was willing to put her trust in our limited abilities which made all the difference. Lastly, as we progressed through this book, it became clear that we simply wanted to record our sincere thanks to the many people who, whatever their background, have come together in our support. The kindness, loyalty and cooperation of a team is indeed the very basis of our present life, and that surely says something about dependence, independence and community.

Foreword

Many changes and new developments affecting the lives of people with handicaps were taking place in Norwich in the late 1960s. When Jack and Margaret Wymer moved into their new flat in 1969 they seemed to symbolise locally the culmination of a period of changing attitudes and new opportunities. Even so, many caring, involved and knowledgeable people found it difficult to believe that they would be able to achieve the degree of independence they were aiming for and have now accomplished.

Knowing what to regard as "normal" is always difficult, but for most of us the ability to exercise control over as much of our own lives as possible, especially our private life, is an essential ingredient of our normality. To be able to exercise choice is vital for life if we are to develop our own potential, but making choices means taking risks. It means risking failure. Society too often wishes, unrealistically, to impose a risk-free environment on people with physical, mental or social handicaps, restricting their lives and limiting their potential development. People in society have difficulty in coping with their feelings whenever risk taking results in hurt or tragedy. But society would be much healthier, in my view, if we could all accept more openly and readily that risk and the independence essential for human dignity are inter-related.

In writing this book and allowing us to share in their experiences, Jack and Margaret Wymer give us all the chance to see that risk, choice and independence are essential elements in the growth of their relationship and their life together. Apart from the significance of this to themselves they have taught the able-bodied something about living. Their greatest achievement, however, is in demonstrating that the apparently impossible can be done, thereby making it harder for society to deny the same opportunity for independence to other people with handicaps.

I regard myself as especially privileged to have known Elizabeth Barnes, the social worker to whom this book is dedicated. She was a woman of remarkable maturity and wisdom. I know that Jack and Margaret Wymer agree with me that their personal achievements in the last ten years are a tribute also to the special combination of faith and realism of Elizabeth Barnes, who risked, in backing the venture initially, the harsh criticism that can be meted out to professionals if failure results in accident or injury. If, as a result of taking this risk, other people with handicaps are enabled to achieve greater independence, she would have felt well rewarded.

GEORGE MEREDITH
Director of Social Services,
Norfolk County Council.

1: It's Merely Routine Now

Jack and I have been married for eleven years. We live happily together, like most other married couples, sharing our daily routine, our joys and our sorrows. But there the similarity ends, for since birth, we have both suffered from Spinal Muscular Atrophy—a slowly progressive disease affecting all the voluntary muscles. Jack and I have never walked, yet our lives at present are all we ever dreamed of.

It is 8 a.m., and the door buzzer penetrates our half-sleep state. Jack fumbles for the plastic tube tucked under his pillow. Snuggled beneath the bedclothes, I hear the bleeps from the box under our bed as Jack activates his "Patient-Operated Selector Mechanism" to release the lock on the front door. Kay, our first helper of the day, enters. We hear the blinds being opened in the living-room, and the clink of milk bottles being carried into the kitchen. Jack's breathing tells me that he is trying to snatch those last few minutes of respite. Luckily, I regain my alertness almost immediately. Glancing round the bedroom. I still cannot take for granted its decor in our own choice of lemon and green. The ceiling track, supporting the electrically-operated hoist, is as familiar and normal to us as any other part of the furniture.

Bright and cheerful, Kay appears in the bedroom doorway. "Hello. Quite cold outside."

Our helpers are just ordinary people from all kinds of backgrounds, but to us they are special. The various payments we hand them never compensate for all the care they show.

Soon, a bowl of water is placed on the bedside cabinet, and my morning wash commences. We exchange tit-bits of information. "Traffic was awful today. Cycling is really dangerous. I shall have to rush off afterwards—I'm house-hunting this morning."

Occasionally, I have to interrupt: "Can you take the towel out of my ears, and say that again, please?"

My own contribution to the conversation may then be interrupted by the flannel passing over my mouth! It is all treated as a matter of course—all part of the process of getting up.

I am almost oblivious to the fact that I am disabled, and unable to move myself to any appreciable degree. I feel so "normal", and to me, my physical condition is more of an inconvenience than a serious disorder. Jack is actually affected to a greater extent, though no such weakness is reflected in his character! As he clings to his semi-consciousness, I am gradually washed and dressed at his side. What good fortune for him that I have to get out of bed first, before he can be rolled over!

Aided by the hoist, I am lowered into my electrically-powered wheelchair, where I sit straight and well, supported by my surgical brace. Special arm-supports give me a greater range of movement for everyday activities. I now position myself at the dressing-table, and do my hair and my make-up, while Jack is being dressed. Conversation on his part usually begins with a few grunts which mean "I don't wanna get up", but within half an hour, he is going through the same procedure with the hoist. Being mobilised in his own powered wheelchair, he starts to whistle, and takes more interest in the conversation!

By this time, I am filling the teapot from the kettle which stands neatly on its pouring stand to save any lifting. I listen from the kitchen as Kay continues with her news and views, while the electric shaver buzzes round Jack's face, carefully avoiding his moustache and long, bushy sideburns. I carry the cereal bowls through on a special wooden tray which has a hundred-and-one other uses during the course of a day, and usually stays on my lap. At about 9.30 a.m., Kay completes her tasks, and we say goodbye and thanks.

Now we are alone. Our attitude changes almost with the

sound of the door being closed. From being accommodating and even entertaining, as one tends to do in company, our own relationship emerges. Without his spectacles, Jack's blue eyes retain a certain sleepy look, which I love to see.

"Morning, dear."

We touch hands, or perhaps give each other a wry smile.

"Had a good night?"

"Must make some phone calls this morning."

Our breakfast of cereals and fruit juice is a leisurely affair, since we can eat only slowly, anyway. And we revel in this quiet part of the day.

Our Home Help makes three visits each week, for a total of five hours. She does the heavier cleaning, and assists with my week's washing. In her chatty, friendly way, she soon learned to give me the scope to do what I can in the way of housework, which must be a difficult assessment to make with each of her various clients.

The next helper we ourselves pay is our mid-day lady, Kathy. Even the half-hour toilet routine is by no means a dull affair, and we soon become involved in hearing yet another of Kathy's comical experiences.

"What do you think happened to me this morning? My ruddy dog pinched my slipper, and buried it in the garden! Got coffee cheap in the Co-op—do you want some? Where are you going today?" And so it goes on.

From mid-day, we are usually left to our own devices, unless we go out anywhere. Our next paid assistant is not due until about 9.30 p.m., when the process of getting to bed takes roughly an hour. But this does not necessarily mean that we will see no one else before then.

When meeting us now for the first time, people often express wonder and amazement at how conveniently organised our lives seem to be.

"It's nice to think 'they' do things like this for people like you."

"I expect 'they' keep an eye on you, though?"

"Still, you don't really have to worry—not like ordinary people, eh?"

We force our smiles, and make non-committal remarks!

However, those who know us well fully realise that what is referred to as 'all this' could hardly be said to have happened overnight! While admitting to a certain amount of good fortune, a high percentage must surely be attributed to hard work and patience—not just on our part, but on that of many others. The good fortune was being given the opportunity of having our own home in the first place. Nevertheless, it was all a gamble. Like most other unprecedented projects, it could not guarantee any lasting results.

But let us look back in time, and see how it all began.

2: Jack Asks Himself—Is This Really Happening?

We first met when I was fifteen, at one of the weekly meetings of the St Raphael Club for disabled people, in Norwich. The Wednesday evening outing was the highlight of my week, being the only real social event I enjoyed. But for Jack, it was not so much an occasion as the breath of life.

His father had died as a POW in the Second World War, when Jack was thirteen years old, and his mother was left struggling to bring up a young family, one of whom, Sheila, was also afflicted with spinal muscular atrophy.

Although Jack's mother had married again many years later, with all the will in the world she could scarcely cope with two handicapped children, and four other daughters as well. There were no hoists or gadgetry in those days, and money was very short. Therefore, she had to steel herself to the fact that she had little chance in her already overburdened existence to give Jack anything like a normal life.

At the age of nineteen, Jack left a special boarding school for disabled boys, and his grandparents, rallying round in the true family way, cared for him for almost a year. Their pre-fabricated bungalow was quite convenient for his invalid chair, and his step-father and uncle helped grandfather on a rota system with local ambulancemen in looking after his needs. Granny, a matronly little woman with red hair, delighted in serving him the food he enjoyed, albeit increasing his waistline! She would knit cardigans for him, and took pride and pleasure in fussing over her grandson, whom she called "my Jackie". Grandfather, for his part, taught Jack the skills of card-playing, and introduced him at the local on Sundays.

Jack was comfortable and well cared for, but he felt that this state of affairs could not last for long.

"I tried not to ask for too much, but I felt a real burden," Jack once told me. "I hated leaving that school—I enjoyed English and Latin. They gave us real hope, there. I even felt I was Someone."

Many years later, Jack learned that when he left that school, his family were given to understand that he would live only about six months—such was the prognosis of the disease in those early days.

In fact, eleven months had passed at the "prefab.", when Granny reluctantly informed Jack that he would be going into hospital.

"Just for a month, to give us a little rest."

"I felt terrible", admitted Jack, "but I could hardly be annoyed, could I? Sitting in that big ward full of old men on the first day, I could smell a mixture of disinfectant and stale urine. I kept asking myself 'Is this really me?' I kept repeating 'I am Jack Wymer' over and over again in my mind, because I couldn't believe it was happening to me."

The family visited him regularly, and after five weeks, Jack began to ask when he was going home again. The question was evaded several times before his mother finally had to break the news.

"I hope you won't mind, but Nanny can't have you back again."

The words were stunning. Jack knew that his grandparents, both in their middle sixties, could not be expected to cope with looking after him indefinitely. But the situation this left him in seemed so unreal. The unimaginable had happened. Jack's confidence took a steep dive. Those on the ward saw only a morose character with a big chip on his shoulder. No one seemed to know or care how unhappy he was. But this earned him a reputation which was noted on his hospital case-sheets. "Doesn't get on with his fellow men."

Jack had been in hospital for three years, when I first met

him at the Club. His short brown hair was dry and flaky from being washed in liquid soap, and not properly rinsed. With his grey flannels and hand-knitted cardigan, Jack already had that "institutional" appearance. It was difficult to describe. Certainly, he was clean and cared for, but somehow, he had a dazed look on his face. His eyes squinted in a pained fashion when viewing something only a short distance away. He thought he needed spectacles, but he "didn't like to trouble anyone". He was playing cards with some older club members, when I remarked to Sheila: "Doesn't your brother look miserable?"

By contrast, at fifteen, I was very naïve and lighthearted. Oh, but how little I knew then! Not that life had been too unkind to me. Doting parents had rather reluctantly parted with me when I was five, to be educated at a school for disabled girls run by a Dominican order of nuns.

I accepted it all, and my interest in the new faces around me helped to compensate for the strange feeling of loneliness I had. We were disciplined in the way of the Church, and even the most disabled amongst us were expected to share in the domestic chores. I well remember being encouraged to clean the hand-basin, polish the boots and shoes, or clean the silver. With only twenty-four girls, aged between five and sixteen, we all received ample care and attention. I cannot recall ever feeling particularly unhappy, except perhaps when I was in bed with nothing to do, or in sick bay recovering from one of the inevitable childhood diseases!

I could not walk, or even crawl very well, but I soon learned the joys of reading. Something of a dreamer, I frequently left the everyday world, either with or without a book! I eagerly devoured stories like *The Water Babies*, *Black Beauty*, *Little Women*, and many more. By the age of ten, I was learning short-hand and typing, and was convinced by the school that this would probably form the basis of my career for later life. Indeed, there was no doubt that this proved to be a good all-round education for me.

3: Illness Brings New Meaning for Me

My education was interrupted shortly afterwards, when I had to leave the safe, disciplined familiarity of the school. My physical condition had worsened if anything, and I had put on weight, to become more or less confined to a wheelchair. The vague diagnosis offered was that I was probably suffering the consequences of poliomyelitis.

My father's army career took him around the country, and he and Mum usually made a point of taking me to visit medical specialists in each area. After one such visit, the Consultant was hopeful that his particular physiotherapy treatment might get me walking.

With no little trepidation, I entered a children's hospital at Bath, but after a year of hard work on everyone's part, there was still no improvement in my condition. What is more, I received no education whatsoever, and had no books with which to amuse myself. The venture was more than an anti-climax to us all, yet it was nobody's fault.

However, my parents now returned to Norwich, their home town, taking me with them. The next step was taken out of our hands, and before long, I was admitted to a children's convalescent home at Great Yarmouth. My experiences there were very unpleasant, and certainly not worth relating. Suffice it to say that much has been written about such places in which mental cruelty was inflicted on young patients by misguided and unhappy individuals. Here, my only education was that unfairness and cruelty did indeed exist in the world. And I still saw no books.

Finally, at thirteen years old, any hope of getting me to walk was abandoned. I arrived home again with my family, now very overweight, and ignorant in many ways, though too knowing in others! I had precious few belongings—just a handbag and a small battered case. There was little opportunity to accumulate possessions in hospitals, and I was now amply accommodated, bed and all, in what had hitherto been called the breakfast room.

Dad had left the army, and was now working as a bus conductor. He found that the shiftwork enabled him to assist Mum in looking after me, and he could also be present when the physiotherapist called to administer my continued treatment.

It was a difficult stage for us all. My brothers Michael and David were seven and six years old respectively, and almost strangers to me. The small council house seemed packed with all of us, compared with the accustomed spaciousness of the hospitals. I became quite hysterical when left alone indoors, and preferred sitting in the garden, even for hours on end.

But gradually, I learned new disciplines, and easily made friends with the neighbours' children. I was even pushed to the cinema on occasions, if wheelchairs were admitted.

My schooling consisted of one two-hour session a week, and the home teacher set me homework for periods in between. But somehow, my thirst for learning had now deserted me. I was more interested in watching games in the park, listening to "pop" music, or hearing intriguing whispers of boy friends from other girls. I was blending nicely into the new domestic scene by now, to the extent of reluctantly darning socks!

As a teenager, life seemed good to me. I was happy in my own way, and the better for being treated as "normal" by the family. I had a deep interest in people, and was quite curious about their lives. My interest in men was non-existent—except in love stories and films. I was blissfully unaware of all those things which I was supposed to be missing in my life.

Through the St Raphael Club, I was now learning to play chess with a young male helper. Len and I became firm friends, but that was as far as it went. Marriage was not for me.

Fortunately for me, I had an optimistic disposition, and was quite easily pleased. I knew no jealousy of my able-bodied friends, and readily accepted that they could have new clothes, while I persevered with my old ones. My parents were far from rich, and Mum had precious few things herself. My friends could earn money—I could not. That was sufficient reason for me. I derived satisfaction from the fact that I was warm, and well fed. What disputes I did have with my parents never concerned new possessions. But I jealously guarded my bed table which held my books and other bits and pieces, hotly insisting that no one should touch them—least of all, my brothers.

"I don't want my things interfered with," I protested.

"They were doing no harm," Mum defended the boys.

"I know, but I want things left alone."

"You must learn to share."

This last rejoinder usually left me red in the face, and I fell sullenly silent.

On other occasions, disputes arose when I would insist as forcibly as possible on going out with my friends, and whatever the weather refusing to have a blanket over my my legs.

"That's for old people in bath chairs," was my indignant reminder.

Indeed. I had my vanity, despite my physical drawbacks. My brown, wavy hair usually behaved well whoever snipped at it, family or friends. I liked it short, as was the trend in those days. With some considerable effort, I would brush it over and over again, secretly admiring the chestnut-coloured highlights. Make-up was beyond my purse, but I enjoyed hearing people say "Isn't she pretty?"

I had become friendly with Jack's sister Sheila on my club nights, when we laughed a lot, and sang around the piano. She told me that it was getting physically more difficult for her to live at home, and she was soon to be admitted to a ward in the same hospital as her brother. At the time, I thought little of it. To me, Jack was still a distant figure in the clubroom, always looking seriously at his playing cards. Sheila always seemed happy, and usually surrounded by boy-friends. If any rivalry existed between us two girls, it was about our appearance only, since I did not feel the need for boy-friends. But I enjoyed hearing about Sheila's amorous exploits!

Vanity was to prove my downfall, however, when during that November I contracted influenza. Going out in the bitter winter evenings wearing just a thin jacket and skirt was asking for trouble. With my history of chest infections, I was taking an unforgivable risk, and Mum despaired of trying to make me see sense. But I had my way.

I can still recall that awful penetrating cold weather. And later that month, 'flu worsened to pneumonia. Modern antibiotics were not readily available then, and by Christmas I was critically ill in hospital.

The night I was rushed into hospital remains a hazy memory. It had been a desperate struggle to keep me alive during the previous few weeks. I could not cough by myself, and Dad had repeatedly turned me face downwards on the bed, performing some kind of artificial respiration. I had to be watched day and night. Poor Mum could not handle my helpless body as easily as Dad could, and at times she was frantic. So it was a great relief to us all when the hospital took over.

I remember that my mother was with me, and I heard the doctor say: "She won't last the night. Better fetch your husband."

Coming to, later on, I was relieved to find myself still in the land of the living, though encased in what is commonly known as an iron lung. I had seen polio victims in these fearsome-looking contraptions many times. The long metal box is connected to an electric pump by means of a large tube at one end, while the patient's head protrudes through a port-hole padded with rubber and cotton wool at the other. Pumping air in and out causes alternate pressure and vacuum which helps the patient's chest to fall and rise in normal breathing action, and various dials are set to regulate air-pressures to the individual breathing rate.

I had seen how these machines could save lives, and I was confident in relying on one now. It felt marvellous to have all the responsibility for breathing taken away. While aware of having blocked lungs, and aches and pains everywhere, I knew that I was not going to die. I beamed the reassurance to my father, sitting near me : "Hello, Dad. I'm going to be all right now."

I shall always remember the visible change which came over Dad's face! The Ward Sister nodded compassionately: "I should go and get some rest now."

During the weeks that followed, I vaguely recall phrases like "collapsed lung", and "postural drainage" being mentioned in my hearing. I was placed with my head and shoulders hanging over the side of the bed, while a patient physiotherapist pounded away on my back. It was a triumph when I could declare to her "I've coughed some up today."

I remember learning to feed myself again, scarcely able to hold the spoon at first.

Gradually, I recovered sufficiently to return home. I was still very weak, weighing under six stone, and uncommonly subdued. Needing most of the time in bed, I did not even care about being kept indoors. I welcomed my own little room again, all neat and clean, with the familiar old bed table still nursing my books and pens and puzzles.

In all, my battle for survival had lasted four months, taking me past my seventeenth birthday. It had been a traumatic experience indeed, yet one which I respected, somehow. A new calm descended upon me. I loved gazing out of my window to the woods bordering on to the back garden. I preferred the birdsong to my radio. As for darning socks, I actually asked for the work, and enjoyed doing it! I rediscovered pleasure in poetry, and found self-expression in writing some of my own. All in all, life had taken on a new meaning, and I valued it wholeheartedly.

4: Getting to Know One Another

Sheila had been in hospital for about a year, when a decision was taken to move the younger disabled elsewhere. The authorities felt that conditions would be better for them in another geriatric hospital just outside the city. Indeed, Sheila was quick to tell me how much nicer the new place was, compared with where she and Jack had been living. She also told me of the Relief Care Scheme, whereby disabled people could be taken into hospital for short stays while families had their holidays.

Coincidentally, my family had received an invitation to stay with some friends in Scotland. I heard Mum and Dad discussing how to cope with getting me and my wheelchair up the stairs to the first-floor flat, but somehow, I did not feel happy with any of the arrangements. Only a few months since my illness, I still tired too easily to do much except live quietly. So, not wishing to offend my parents, I gently told them what Sheila had said. I pointed out how nice it would be for Sheila and me to have a couple of weeks together. What is more, my family would find it easier to go sightseeing without me.

My parents agreed quite readily, and I wrote to the hospital myself for an admittance during that August 1955. So it was arranged. We had no car of our own, so I had to travel by ambulance. Little did I realise what a great effect that short journey would have on my whole life!

The hospital had been converted from a large old house, formerly owned by a local business man. It stood amidst beautiful gardens and rambling grounds, which included a pleasant little lake secluded by trees and bushes. Indeed, the setting could scarcely have been more inviting, under the circumstances. The elderly infirm patients occupied the two upper floors. However, Jack and three other young men were privileged to live downstairs, at least for the time being.

Their bedroom, with its panelled walls and concealed lighting around the ornate ceiling, seemed ideal. French doors opened on to a covered balcony, which in turn overlooked sunken gardens. During the day, Jack and his friends would sit in the bay window of a larger room, where Sheila and I joined them.

I began to see Jack in a new light. He was always doing funny impressions of people, and making witty puns. He made me laugh, and I began to enjoy his company. He was warming towards me. We frequently asked to be put side by side at the end of the balcony, so as to be alone together. We got to know each other a little better every day. Jack admitted much later that he was feeling more and more attracted to me.

At twenty-five, he was much wiser than I, but said that he liked my commonsense manner. He had usually found girls to be rather frivolous. We talked and talked about everything. I received no direct compliments for Jack was not gifted with a tongue for flattery, but what impressed me about him was his steady acceptance of life in general. I was never really aware of his handicapped state: only of the warmth in his eyes as they met mine. My heart seemed to flip, and I blushed easily. Secretly, he enjoyed this new found power, which previously he had thought he lacked!

We still remember when Jack daringly touched my hand for the first time, and I snatched it away, amazed by his brashness! We have often smiled since when comparing the incident with modern-day standards!

But to us, those feelings being aroused were strong and real. Whereas before I had only been amused by my friends' excited chat about boy-friends, now I could understand the full meaning behind it. I had mixed with boys before, making one or two close friends, but nothing was ever as exciting as this.

Jack was the nicest person to be with. He had the kind of dependable character that I liked, yet possessed an audacity which as time passed was to capture me completely. But for now, all it did was to play havoc with my emotions, and make the world seem a much happier place.

Leaving Jack at the end of that fortnight was to be the first of many painful partings. At home that night, I cried. But I cherished the wonderful secret of our friendship.

After a few days, I calmly informed my parents that I, too, wanted to leave home, and live in the hospital! Not revealing my true reasons, I simply said: "I may as well go now while I want to, as later in life, when it could be harder."

Mum and Dad were clearly shaken by my request, scarcely knowing how to cope. Initially, they seemed to accept the idea, perhaps hoping that I would change my mind. But as my plans reached some conclusion, my father became very determined. "At seventeen, you are not allowed to make those kind of decisions. When you're twenty-one, you can do as you wish. But until then, I'm keeping you under this roof."

I was angry, and miserable. Jack's reaction to it all, as revealed in his letters, was more philosophical. He consoled me by saying that it was for the best. "You're better off living at home, really."

I settled down gradually, living from one letter to the next, as we each wrote every other day. It was an unusual courtship, indeed, but we learned a lot about one another, and thoroughly enjoyed it.

5: Regretfully Accepting Our Limitations

As if the year had not been eventful enough, there was more to come. In October, my mother revealed that she was expecting a baby. We were all thrilled. The fact that she was nearly thirty-seven years old did not seem to matter.

Our pleasure was shortlived. By November, it became obvious from the yellow tinge to her skin, and the slowness of her pace, that Mum was very unwell. Infective hepatitis was diagnosed, and she was confined to bed, while we anxiously awaited her recovery.

There was no improvement by Christmas, and on Boxing Day, an ambulance took her into hospital—to the same ward, in fact, where I had been only twelve months previously.

Somehow, we all muddled through at home. I was put in charge of the housekeeping, since Dad was at work, and my brothers, now aged ten and eleven, were at school. A Sister of a Catholic order came in at midday, and again at teatime, to attend my needs, and to prepare meals for us all.

It seemed an empty house without Mum. I missed her busying around, chatting incessantly, and making the house seem so alive. I was faced with new responsibilities, like making sure the food cupboard was well stocked, arranging the menus, doing Dad's sandwiches for work the next day, or just listening to the boys' little troubles. It was a bad time for them, too. Dad worked from 8 a.m. until 6.30 p.m. Then he would visit Mum. By the time he returned, Michael and David were washed and ready for bed.

Sometimes, I tried to surprise Dad by coping with the washing up myself. My brothers often preferred to bring me a bowl of water and all the crockery on to my bed, than do the job themselves in the kitchen!

I rarely got dressed and put in my wheelchair in those days. It was warmer in bed, and I had been used to coping with everything from that position for some time now. Besides, it made life so much easier for Dad.

However, I did get up on Wednesday evenings, for my weekly outing to the club, where I could sit with Jack. I drew great strength from our meetings, though at home I mentioned little about them.

Mum's condition worsened. The doctors wanted to terminate the pregnancy. They felt that this was hampering her recovery. Mum firmly refused. Her religious beliefs would not allow such action. Then it was decided to perform an exploratory operation. My father broke the news to me with profound seriousness, and added: "They now suspect cancer."

It was a terrible blow. Somehow, I felt both grown-up and yet still a child, all at the same time. Dad looked tired and drawn. My heart ached for him, though I could find no words to console him.

The operation took place in February. It was a grey day, which only added to the sadness, and I spent the entire day thinking about it all. If only I could just get to a telephone on my own!

At long last, Dad returned home looking extremely relieved. There was definitely no cancer. "Mum won't get over the liver infection while she's pregnant," explained Dad. "She could have another handicapped child, because they can't see how a baby can survive and develop properly under the circumstances. But Mum won't agree to end the pregnancy, and I can't persuade her, so we'll just have to wait and see."

My eighteenth birthday was due on March 19th, and Mum was eager to be home for it. She was still being nursed on a fat-free diet, and needed regular dressings on the operation wound, which in her poor condition would not heal. There was no question of her doing anything at home. But a Home Help was allowed in, and Mum promised to obey all the rules.

It was lovely to have her home again. Her hair was still a grey colour, and her face was yellow and lined. But she was happy just to move around slowly, and organise a few things. She spent a lot of time sitting at the end of my bed, knitting things for the baby that she was still determined to have.

Dad looked much happier, grateful to have Mum around, however little she could do for him. I never heard him complain, though there cannot be many men who have had to attend so willingly to all a daughter's physical needs, as well as help their wife into the bath and up to bed every night after a day's work.

Our cosy routine continued for several weeks, before it was again rudely interrupted. One Saturday night late in March, Mum showed signs of going into labour, and was taken to hospital again. This time I would have to go away somewhere, too, and a neighbour would have Michael and David after school until late evening. These new arrangements were thought preferable to the way we had all struggled on before.

Secretly, I hoped my journey would take me to Jack. But my parents remained very non-committal on the subject, and I feared that they would not allow us to be together in that way again. All I knew was that I would be going wherever there was a vacancy.

Dad had said his goodbyes before leaving for work, and I was left ready in my wheelchair, with suitcase at hand. I prayed silently to myself "Please let it be with Jack." It was the contact of our letters, and our weekly meetings in that crowded clubroom, which had given meaning to my life all this time. I never discussed what he meant to me with any of my friends or family. So impossible seemed our situation, that it appeared to invite only ridicule.

How I needed him now. The reassuring smile, and the warmth of his hand, would have eased this empty feeling so much.

When my transport arrived, I could not bring myself to ask where the driver was taking me. But as I feared, it was not in the direction I wanted. Later on, I learned that my destination was a hospital some sixteen miles outside Norwich. My heart sank, and I fought back the tears. I still clung to a vain hope that I could get to the club to see Jack.

On my arrival, I put on a brave front, and cheerfully greeted the staff. My room was rather pleasant. I had the luxury of my own room, with a lovely view of the hospital grounds. My first thought was to write to Jack, and then I asked if I might telephone the club president. Puzzled glances were exchanged amongst the nurses.

"It's against hospital rules for patients to use the office phone, and we haven't got a public call box."

The ominous tone of voice seems an ever present part of the "invisible restraint" in such places. But after some consultation, I was allowed to telephone, to see if my transport could be arranged for club night. Of course, the answer was a firm but apologetic "No."

Meanwhile, Jack knew nothing of these latest developments. My letter had not reached him, and he was still expecting to see me at the club. We were both sadly disappointed.

For a time, Jack and I corresponded as usual, but suddenly there seemed little to write about from my end. We felt strangely disillusioned, concluding that we had absolutely no control over our own destiny. This limited friendship was all we could ever expect. Handicapped people were moved around like pawns, to comply with the wishes of everyone else. They had no say in what mattered to them.

That was how things were—and there was no prospect of any change. To separate us in this way, without a thought for our feelings, was callous, but we had to go where we were put. What was the use of pledging ourselves to one another, when it was obvious that we each needed a *normal* partner?

This was Jack's bitter reaction, anyway. I only felt more and more depressed. I would have favoured hanging on to what little we had, however remote, rather than a complete break. But our letters ceased. I felt too low to argue at all. Now I knew what real loneliness meant.

The hospital staff were kind to me, probably thinking that my silence and private tears were for my family. I was dressed every day, and sat in my wheelchair. My needs were few. I liked having a pen and paper, and a small mouth-organ which I was learning to play. My pleasure was enhanced by sitting in the garden when the sun shone.

In fact, six weeks dragged by in this manner. I received one or two short letters from my mother, but that was the only family contact I could reasonably expect at such a distance. Slowly, I became conditioned to this comfortable though dull existence. Goodness knew how long it would last. If my mother did not survive, would it last for ever? I banished the thought quickly.

When Sunday came, it looked like being just the same as any other day to me. My one consolation was that the sun was shining brightly. So I could not believe my eyes when suddenly I saw Dad approaching from the driveway! His face was bright and beaming, and I knew that it must be good news, which he had cycled all the way to bring me.

"You have another brother," were his first words, adding meaningfully, "And he's all pink, too."

The baby weighed only four pounds, which meant that it might be a week or so before he was allowed home. Mum had named him Gerard, after the Patron Saint of Mothers-to-be, in whom she had put so much faith.

My homecoming seemed too good to be true. That bleak day of my departure was thankfully fading in the light of Mum's already apparent improvement. We soon settled into a new routine, which now included the baby. It was a great pleasure for me to feed him, and play with him on my bed, where he nestled very often.

This added interest in my life helped to numb any feelings I nurtured for Jack. But there were sad reminders of our happy times as I arrived at the club each week. The helpers joked good-naturedly as they assumed that we still wanted to sit side by side. Now it was slightly embarrassing when I had to ask to be moved away from Jack, and it became obvious that there was a change in our relationship!

We both realised that the mutual feelings between us were still strong, but I tried to take Jack's advice.

"Better for you to mix with other people," he said.

But I could find no company like Jack's.

6: Jack's Despair and Determination

Meanwhile, Jack's life continued somewhat drearily. He was always seeking to occupy his time usefully, and if such occupation should bring him some monetary reward, then all the better! Though to what purpose he should be earning, as yet he knew not.

Jack's endeavours stemmed from those early days in hospital when, again through the club, he had obtained a little outwork from a local cracker-making factory. This involved glueing together the various parts of the coloured outer wrapping, and called for a good deal of precision. The work was prepared flat in readiness for feeding into a machine which would roll and fill each cracker to completion. Jack's limited arm movements could produce only five and a half gross in a week, and at 11p. a gross it was hard earned money.

His first consignment was rejected, but he soon became suitably proficient, and found the work enjoyable.

When he was moved to the second hospital, Jack's routine was disrupted and the cracker-making was forgotten. But a visiting Arts and Crafts teacher brought a new impetus to his creative ability, and he began drawing his own Christmas cards and writing the appropriate verses in a neat italic script. So successful were the cards that he could not meet the demand.

The teacher also rekindled Jack's interest in music, and taught him to write the notation to short pieces which he was already playing on his harmonica. Daringly, he was soon submitting his own songs to London publishers in beautifully written manuscript, complete with melody line and lyrics.

Alas, the rejection slips came back with discouraging regularity. But Jack persevered for ten years, before finally giving up hope of succeeding in so competitive a field.

After the first year, Jack and I found ourselves writing to each other again, especially when there seemed something important to say, for we were still good friends. One letter from Jack has stuck in my memory.

"I feel so low that I just had to write. We've all been moved from the ground floor to an attic room. Without warning, our things were being taken towards the lift. Something was said about the builders coming in to make some alterations. . . .

As I read on, my heart went out to him.

". . . . The three of us are in this small room—it's about ten feet square, with a slanted ceiling. We have our beds and our lockers, and a table around which we all sit in our wheelchairs. There's so little space, that if we're not placed in correct order, we won't all fit in properly. I have to sit with my back to the window, but anyway, we can only see the tree-tops. The only change of scenery we have is in the mornings when we're put in the day-room with the old men while our room is cleaned. . . ."

Poor Jack was back where he started: back to the too-familiar smell of stale urine and the weird sounds of senility and wandering minds, which he thought had been left behind. He even admitted to weeping in the depths of despair, and wrote several letters imploring the powers-that-be to improve this demoralising situation. But no one seemed to have the authority to rectify it.

I felt desperately sad, and so very helpless. I remembered the spacious accommodation Jack enjoyed when I had spent my two weeks there. I was bitterly angry at such blatant inconsideration. It seemed that Jack and his pals were shut away without a second thought. They were not even allowed downstairs unaccompanied for safety reasons, and I know that Jack, for one, enjoyed the gardens so much.

Once so appreciative of his improved conditions, Jack was

now more bitter than ever about the way he had been treated. I tried to console him in my return letter, but could only admit to sharing his disgust. I failed to understand why I should have the good fortune of a secure family home, while Jack led a prison-like existence. But in spirit, I drew closer to him than ever.

A fresh determination then set him on another profitable hobby, making dressing-table mats. The work was self-taught from someone else's original idea, and involved stretching threads across a wooden frame, and knotting at each intersection. Trimmed round the edges, the article was completed by teaseling the frayed ends with a wire brush. The orders came rolling in at 37½p. for a set of three! Producing two sets each week, Jack made a profit of some 45p. equal to the weekly pocket money then afforded to the disabled in hospital by the National Assistance Board!

Satisfied with his returns, Jack ignored the sore finger which resulted from pulling the thread so tightly. Never too keen to part with his hard-earned cash, he turned to buying Savings Stamps, and was content to feel that one day, something better must materialise.

Jack began to strike up a mutual understanding with some of the staff, and two or three would visit the tiny attic room during their lunch break to laugh and joke with him and his fellow patients. Warmer days meant short excursions into the garden. And occasionally Jack managed to persuade one of the girls to take him for a walk outside the hospital grounds, and along the country roads. He relished the change of scenery, as well as the female company.

Outings generally were all too infrequent, but faithfully, the weekly club evenings continued. Then trips to the Norwich City football ground became more regular, as a Scout Master organised his senior scouts to push Jack in his wheelchair for the two miles distance. The Scout Master, Alec, was to become a close friend. He used his works van for taking Jack out and about, and by this convenient means Jack was able to visit his mother for the day, or attend an occasional concert.

Jack's optimism was slowly returning. The threads of goodwill were beginning to weave a pattern into the fabric of his life. Indeed, these were some indication of the subsequent wealth of kindness, friendship and support which has accompanied both of us through to the present day.

No small part of this pattern was a new member of the hospital staff—a nineteen-years-old male nurse named Trevor. He learned to look after Jack very well, and a lasting friendship began.

7: We Pledge Ourselves

The year 1959 was to prove an important one in our story. The family were all coping well, and our routine was running smoothly. I was happy with my life, and enjoyed being able to contribute to the domestic scene in little ways which were useful when Mum was ill. Baby Gerard was now three, and I delighted in entertaining him for a large part of my day by singing to him or reading stories.

My parents now felt ready for another holiday, and planned to have a couple of weeks at the coast. They seemed happy for me to make arrangements to go into the hospital again, knowing that Sheila and I were still good company for each other, and feeling that perhaps Jack did not hold the same attraction for me now!

I found many alterations at the hospital, and not all of them were structural. Sheila and I were on the big ward wih the old ladies, whilst Jack and his pals were on the floor above us. However, we were all allowed to watch television together in the evenings. It was certainly not the pleasant situation we had all enjoyed before. But it was to prove to be the renewal of all those past wonderful feelings.

Jack and I had a mutual interest in the game of chess. Insisting that we could not possibly concentrate on playing in the television room, he cleverly contrived to have us put in a smaller room which was otherwise vacated for the evening. There we set up our chess board, thankful to be alone and quiet.

We spent several evenings in this way. We played a lot of chess, and did a great deal more talking. I am pleased to say that not all the moves were made on the chess board. Jack began to re-open what I had assumed was a closed door. He admitted to feeling the same about me, despite all his attempts to change things between us.

"I know you haven't changed, so can we start again?" he asked. "Let's take what we have, and let the future take care of itself."

I was now much more aware, and even slightly sceptical. I wondered just where this new gambit would lead us. I wanted to be persuaded, yet doubted whether I could be. So many mixed feelings tormented me. Sitting either side of our table, we could not even touch one another to be reassured.

I made no definite promises, but those two weeks left me with much to think about. The stalemate position no longer existed for me. In our hearts, we were quietly happy. We had decided independently that we were meant for each other, but were still too wary to disclose our feelings fully.

Our letters increased. The pen became the instrument of expressing our love. It mattered not how limited we were now. We would gratefully accept what we had, and without question.

One person who was sympathetic to our cause was Trevor. He occasionally visited me, and would tell me of his own plans. His girlfriend, Freda, was also disabled. She lived forty miles from Norwich, and therefore Trevor could only get to see her fortnightly. When he knew about Jack, he offered to take me to see him, fully realising our problems.

With no transport of our own, complicated arrangements included catching two buses, and another half-mile walk at the other end of the journey. Trevor had to lift me on to the bus, and then fold my portable wheelchair to carry that on as well. For a faster change-over, it was sometimes possible to perch me on a convenient wall nearby, and to have my chair folded in readiness when the bus arrived!

Trevor's unselfish attitude over these fortnightly visits always impressed us. He would leave us sitting together, supposedly watching television, in the day-room, which was otherwise deserted by late afternoon, whilst he diplomatically disappeared to the floor below to sit and talk with Sheila!

Jack and I enjoyed these meetings, which became our most important times together. We got as close to each other as our wheelchairs permitted, with no fear of prying eyes. We would sit with our heads together, and talk about what we would do if circumstances were different. Not that we were ever unhappy at the apparent hopelessness of our situation. The mutual warmth and strength of our companionship was a gift which many did not possess, and it could never be overshadowed in any way. It was wonderful enough in itself to have someone to share with, someone to confide in—someone to love.

About this time, there was talk of a new purpose-built home for younger disabled people. In fact, it had been rumoured for about ten years, but now a site was secured near the city centre and building was well under way. On three occasions, Alec took Jack to see the work in progress.

"I don't know if I'll be able to qualify," Jack told me. "I've heard that one must be able to work, and we've got to have an IQ test or something. Doubt whether I'll be one of the chosen few," he added in a more serious note.

But fortunately for us, Jack was selected for the new home.

8: A New Home, a New World for Jack

On Friday July 15th 1960, Jack and Sheila were transferred to the new unit. Just the two of them from that hospital were chosen, and Jack was a little disturbed that his fellow patients had not been accepted. In fact both he and his sister were asked by the authoritities to delay the move until the new home agreed to take all of them, but he had waited for such a chance so long that, despite many guilty feelings, he dared not refuse what could be his only opportunity. Therefore, Jack and Sheila were required formally to discharge themselves from the hospital.

This new home represented a different concept in accommodation for severely disabled people, and when Jack and his sister arrived, they were delighted with everything. Eleven double bedrooms and eight single were arranged around three sides of a courtyard, while the sitting-room, dining-room and kitchen completed the rectangle. It was sheer luxury to have separate rooms for each function. Being got up for breakfast and allowed to remain out of bed until late evening were just two long forgotten privileges. Rules and regulations in the hostel were almost negligible. Residents and friends were free to come and go at will.

"Fancy!" I reported to my mother, "Fancy! they even have electric wheelchairs at that new place!"

Jack had been allowed to borrow such a powered chair, and it made all the difference in the world to him. His whole outlook changed. He had never been able to propel himself in an ordinary wheelchair, as I was able to do with difficulty in those days. Now, the ability to move freely at the touch of a switch immediately broadened his horizons. He was able at liberty to pass from one room to the next; to wander into the courtyard for catching the sun; to go and socialise with a new resident. Mobility in itself was sheer enjoyment. Never before had Jack been so punctual for his meals, despite jolting the table, often violently, in the process!

He was more than a little scared when first put in control of his powered chair, and needed all the wide corridors and spaciousness of the hostel for practising. Hitherto there had always been someone behind him to guide his push-chair, and to stop it as necessary. Now he must do these things himself. Learning angles of approach, and gauging widths of clearance and braking distances, are skills normally acquired from childhood. For Jack, at the age of thirty, the discovery was far more exciting!

No wonder he began to develop that air of confidence which I loved to see in him. He enjoyed gazing out of the windows and observing signs of everyday life. He watched the comings and goings of the tradesmen, housewives hanging out their washing, the children playing in the street, men returning home from work in the evening. He got to know and speak to many of them, as he sat outside. He now felt a part of the community.

In a central part of the city, more opportunities present themselves. Jack's outings increased. He became even more of a familiar face at the football ground, when Trevor's brother-in-law Mike took on the job of pushing him the shorter distance. More concerts and cinema trips became available.

"It's like being introduced to society!" he laughingly said.

In all, Jack had spent ten years on hospital geriatric wards, and now needed time to take stock of his new life. At first, he did little else except letter-writing. Getting used to his chair and to new people and surroundings was quite enough.

But inevitably he was soon to start forming his own disciplines and hobbies. His new venture was assembling costume jewellery. This craft proved to be his most successful enterprise in every way. It involved mail-order purchasing of the component parts, and setting the polished stones into the ready-made mounts. Both natural gems and ordinary chatons were used, and a clear adhesive made the work easy for Jack to handle. Satisfaction and creativity came in the colours and pattern chosen, and brooches, bracelets, pendants and ear-rings made a fine display for prospective customers.

Alec had acquired an old school desk for Jack to work on, and set it up in his corner of the hobbies room. Jack was busy once more. Every morning after breakfast he would drive his chair from the table, through the television lounge, to take up his position in the hobbies room. There he would work until lunch-time. In the afternoons he allowed himself a break, either sitting outside or watching the world go by from the window. Jack relied on his own salesmanship for disposing of his jewellery, with an occasional sale organised by the visiting handicrafts teacher.

Jack's settled state had a good effect on me. If he was happy, then so was I. We still took each day as it came, not daring to look too far ahead. But best of all, transport permitting, I could arrange to spend a whole day at a time with Jack. And many Saturdays saw my brothers, sixteen-year-old Michael, and David now fifteen, pushing me almost three miles to the hostel. There was no fun in it for them, and their willingness to help could never have been accounted for by the small payments I offered. But the arrangement sufficed for quite a long time.

My own home routine was quietly organised. It still suited me to remain in my high bed for most days. I enjoyed an early start to my day, when I would gaze out of the window to the woods bordering on our back garden. Once Dad had attended to my needs, and sat me up in a well-balanced position, I could get on with my tasks. The bed itself presented an ideal work surface, with space enough to spread my things around. My writing materials, books, socks to darn, and other mending jobs all found a place. Even the sewing machine was often accommodated on my bed! I preferred to be organised for the whole day, and planned everything accordingly. Usually, my brothers would fetch me the necessary things before dashing off to school.

I learned to use Mum's electric sewing machine by depressing the foot-pad with my elbow. Besides coping with a good deal of family mending, I started to produce a few aprons for sale, as well as making myself a blouse or two.

Utilising the surface of my bed even further, there seemed scope enough to attempt anything. Plaster moulds were very messy, and not at all successful. I enjoyed painting the finished articles, but was often disappointed when peeling away the rubber mould to find disfiguring flaws. However, I did succeed in launching a new project when I began to make model ships. Assembling plastic kits of many famous old sea-going craft, I delighted in painting them to the smallest detail, and completed the models with intricate cotton rigging. The *Santa Maria* was the most popular with my customers, selling at 25p. and making me all of 10p. profit!

These hobbies were self-taught. But there was soon to be another, which turned out to be my favourite—patchwork. Our needlework teacher was very strict, but I always found hand-sewing relaxing and rewarding. Sheila was also in the needlework class, formed from the teacher's best pupils, and we all worked together on a huge patchwork quilt.

We received 4p. an hour for our labours!

9: Highlights and Holidays

Of all our various interests, there was one which created a lot of fun, as well as encouraging us to move out even further into the community—harmonica playing. With Jack playing the bass chord harmonica and generally arranging the tunes for us, Sheila taking the melody and me doing the harmony, we practised whenever possible. Eventually we could make quite a good sound! Pop songs of the day could often be simplified to suit our group. To add variety, Jack would arrange one of his own compositions.

Thus we formed our group called "The Harmonicas Three". We got ourselves many bookings around the clubs and pubs, played at garden fetes and charity shows, and entered local talent contests. We even did a broadcast on local radio.

It was essential to have our own transport for getting to the various venues, and Jack decided to cash all his Savings Stamps and buy an old van for £45. Dad had been looking into the possibilities for us, and he and Mum were willing to share the costs of tax and insurance. Dad could use the van for work, and it might prove useful in many ways. And we certainly got around.

Squeezed into the back of the old van, we must have presented a funny sight as the long wooden ramp was put into position for our exit. We earned three guineas for each gig, and put some money towards travelling expenses, and some towards new instruments. Very rarely did we keep any for ourselves. We became quite well known, and enjoyed it all. Dad was most tolerant. No doubt there were many times when he would rather not have been dragged out to drive us to some remote venue. Nevertheless, he came.

The bright lights seemed to flicker more often now. Jack

and I both felt that this was the zenith of everything. We were able to meet more often. Our social life was expanding. We were grateful for what we had found between us. Gradually, we learned more and more about each other. We knew what we liked—and we liked what we knew. Our pleasures were small and simple. We talked about the past. And the future? Oh, if only we had lots of money . . . !

Holidays were times enjoyed by "normal people". Certainly I never gave them a thought. Jack was always reluctant to have strangers looking after him, so he too dismissed the holiday idea. However, the club had considered for some time that disabled people should know the fun and freedom of a holiday. The idea was certainly new, but soon gained support from other sources.

Therefore, special arrangements were made by the club, and disabled people were allocated a separate week at a holiday camp in Gorleston. Jack, Sheila and I took our chance gladly. Trevor was amongst the band of voluntary helpers, which made things easier from Jack's point of view. But the biggest attraction was that Jack and I would be together for a whole week!

To make our holiday more fun, Jack managed to borrow a powered chair for me to use. Thus, for the first time, we could wander off together along the garden paths, around the tennis courts and down to the sports field and swimming pool. We dutifully entered a few games competitions, but mostly we would steal away to a secluded corner of the camp. A favourite spot was the swimming pool area, where we would sit for long periods in the sun, with our heads close together.

These romantic moments were often interrupted by fits of laughter, as we recalled some mishap with my chair. I was experiencing the same difficulties as Jack had at first, only more so. On one occasion the front wheel hit a stone, and the steering handle went out of control. I slid forward precariously in the chair, which proceeded to go into an alarming spin.

Jack called to a Spanish waiter for help, positioned his own chair to prevent mine spinning round, and eventually explained to the waiter how to make me comfortable again.

It was more embarrassing than frightening, I do believe. As it was, there were the usual insinuations about women drivers. Even Jack, in his most understanding way, had to admit that he had "never known a driver to manœuvre so much, and finish up in the same place!"

Jack was fascinated with the camp's Variety Shows every evening, for he had long had a passion for Showbiz. He was interested in all aspects of staging concerts, and was often left in wonderment at a particular musical virtuoso. Jack was enjoying this holiday more than he thought was possible.

Afterwards, we wandered outside alone. Taking a kiss beneath the night sky was simply perfect. Must we say Goodnight? Why cannot every day be like today . . . ?

We even stretched our waking hours by arranging secret meetings in Jack's chalet. We felt it was a pity to let all our evenings come to an unceremonious halt at 10 p.m., though we usually accepted it, realising that the hard-worked helpers needed a rest. But at his own suggestion, Trevor would sometimes return after his duties to take me to Jack's chalet, where I could stay until about midnight.

Stealing into my chalet at half past ten, Trevor would whisk me away, with trousers and coat slipped over my pyjamas. In no time at all, I was being raced through the chill night air in an old push-chair. Trevor was out of breath in his haste to get me there unnoticed. Fortunately, only a few last-minute stragglers roamed the camp. They must have been puzzled by the emergency dash of a bundle of clothes in a wheelchair!

Jack had a chalet to himself, and he sat propped up in bed, waiting for me. I sat somehow across his lap. There we stayed, quietly enjoying our mutual embraces. Our secret added to the excitement. We talked in whispers, growing steadily more dozy, yet still not wanting to relinquish the night.

Meanwhile, Trevor was at one of the usual helpers' parties, perhaps with Freda. But even she did not know why Trevor would suddenly leave.

"I've just got a little job to do. Be back in a minute."

It was sometimes one o'clock when I was returned to my own chalet, not even waking Sheila, who promised not to tell anyway. The helpers could never understand why I was so sleepy next morning!

It was no wonder we felt so sad at the end of our holiday, which was to become an annual event for several years to come.

10: Sheila Dies

Trevor and Freda were married in June 1962. I was pleased to attend that simple but memorable ceremony in the picturesque village church. They had bought a house in Norwich, and soon, Jack and I were being invited round. With help from Trevor's sisters, we often spent a couple of days and nights at a time there. Those marvellous times did much to bring us closer together. We loved the homely atmosphere, and the four of us were firm friends. Jack and I became familiar with the domestic scene, obviously geared to the capabilities of a disabled housewife. But even with severe arthritis, Freda was far more capable than I.

The next two years passed by in the same steady pattern. We were not envious of Trevor's and Freda's situation, for we realised that with an able-bodied partner, most things were possible. For us, it was different. But we had our day-dreams!

Sheila was also enjoying her limited life. She liked a drink, relished her food, and smoked a few cigarettes. Besides her needlework, she did beautiful crocheting. She had a pleasant singing voice, and often obliged with songs at parties or at church services. Everyone knew her as "The girl with red hair, and a lovely voice."

Then one weekend, Sheila had arranged to go out for two days in succession. On the second evening, she returned home unable to sit up properly, and too floppy to control her powered chair. At first, it was simply assumed that she was drunk. But her violent headaches persisted, and eventually the doctor was called.

There was no alarm, at least as far as Jack was concerned. We always knew that Sheila was never as fit even as ourselves. She had a kidney disorder, which led to high blood pressure, and this had caused her many bouts of illness. But she always fought back, often making quite remarkable recoveries.

But Jack's complacency was completely shattered when the doctor revealed that in fact Sheila had suffered a stroke, and was critically ill.

Sheila's mother was summoned, and both she and Jack watched and waited by the bedside. They hated seeing Sheila in so much pain, and were relieved when the doctor paid a second visit with an injection.

After a time, Mother said, "There. She's resting now. Perhaps she'll feel better in the morning.

It was all too much for Jack, and tears rolled down his cheeks, as he sobbed out, "I'm afraid she's not going to get better."

The vigil was kept until the staff persuaded Jack, for his own sake, to go to bed.

Sheila died in the early hours of November 4th, 1964—just a few weeks before her twenty-eighth birthday.

It was a great shock, and attending her funeral later that week seemed unreal to both of us.

Sheila was not the first to die, and obviously would not be the last. The hostel now housed many young disabled people with similarly serious conditions. Ultimately, we all had to accept our own vulnerability.

Slowly, the loss sank in. That our harmonica trio no longer existed was of least consequence. Jack and I went mechanically about fulfilling our two outstanding bookings, but it could never be the same again, and we arranged no more. A part of us had gone which nothing could replace.

11: Facing Jack's Own Vulnerability

A lively personality such as Sheila's was deeply missed at the hostel, and several months passed in strange sobriety. Respiratory infections were also causing serious concern from time to time. I began to get a morbid obsession about Jack's state of health, and was anxious each time he developed the slightest cold.

Yet it was to be the most unsuspected episode which shook me rigid.

We were having breakfast with Trevor and Freda, when I saw Jack gulp. He calmly announced, "I think I'm going to choke."

A piece of bacon had stuck in his windpipe.

Trevor thumped him on the back, and twisted him and turned him all ways to try and dislodge the bacon piece. Jack's mouth would not open wide enough to get a finger down the throat. His face went red, then blue, and all colours, but from the awful noise he made it appeared that he was getting a little air. Trevor picked him up bodily, and turned him upside down in the hope that gravity would help to release the blockage. We all remained deadly calm.

Freda tapped her walking-stick on the wall, and the neighbour was soon telephoning 999. Jack's eyes were staring glassily. I could only look on helplessly.

The ambulance arrived, and the attendants saw Trevor still desperately struggling to keep Jack alive. They shook their heads hopelessly. Trevor wasted no time in carrying Jack into the ambulance, still whooping for breath.

All this had seemed an eternity, yet it lasted barely fifteen minutes. Freda and I could do nothing except wait.

Jack's chair remained in the corner looking empty and forlorn, and echoing exactly how I felt inside. We both said very little. I was fully convinced that Jack would not recover from this incident. All routine was forgotten, and we just waited in silence.

It was two hours before Trevor returned. His face showed a broad grin, and I was immediately reassured that Jack was all right. Only then could I cry—from sheer relief.

Trevor told me that, though a tracheotomy tray had been prepared, it had fortunately not been needed. A "sucker" tube had sufficed. Apparently, Jack was soon back to his old wisecracking self! "Phew! That saved my bacon, didnt it?"

What Trevor did not reveal was that Jack had broken down crying for awhile, so terrifying had been the experience.

Later that afternoon, I went down to the hostel, and could hardly believe it had happened at all. Jack looked so normal, though his throat was still sore. We both felt subdued, and were reluctant to talk about it for some time.

The experience had proved a great shock to Jack. It seemed significant that before long he was suffering many minor infections, and a recurring bladder disorder was becoming more uncomfortable.

He seemed to feel the cold more, and often had a higher than normal temperature. Despite having a good doctor, Jack was still reluctant to bother anyone, and often suffered too long without treatment. His sense of humour was less apparent than usual, and he would lapse into long, gloomy silences.

It was during one of these indifferent spells that he was invited to my home for the day. My parents had long accepted the obvious permanence of our friendship. But another daunting experience was to beset us on that Sunday.

Jack had taken some tablets for his urine infection, when soon afterwards his normally rubicond face turned ashen. He said that his heart felt "funny", and that he felt dizzy and numb. I was holding his hand, which was suddenly hot and clammy. We were all puzzled, and decided to call the doctor.

A locum arrived who knew nothing about Jack, and suggested that he might have been drinking. By now, Jack had begun to talk loudly, and to inform us all that he was dying. He insisted that I should take care of his purse. In my own mind, I was convinced that he was having a nervous breakdown.

Unable to decide what was wrong, the doctor advised that Jack should be taken back to the hostel. I asked Dad to take me as well, but he refused, saying that it would be unwise since there was nothing I could do. So once again I was left waiting and wondering.

How I wished I had a telephone. How I wished that I could go somewhere quiet. But family life hustled and bustled on around me, and I kept my own feelings bottled up inside. If only I did not always have to put up a brave front. But it seemed the only way.

Dad returned. He told me that Jack was put to bed, and that a consultant had been summoned. Again, I resigned myself, thoughtfully turning Jack's purse over and over in my hands. Plans started to formulate in my mind. I must visit him tomorrow. Trevor will take me—his day off from work. But how shall I get a message to him? I know—ring him at work straightaway.

I asked Dad if he would go down to the telephone kiosk on the corner, and make the call for me. He duly complied, and I began to relax.

"Please let Jack be all right," was my silent prayer. But to those around me, I remained quiet.

As if in answer to my prayer, Alec was suddenly at the door! By chance, he had called at the hostel and heard about Jack's "attack". He had waited to see at first hand the results of the consultant's injection. Jack had become calmer, it seemed, and was soon back to normal.

Alec asked if there was anything he could do.

"Let Margaret know I'm all right now. I know she'll be worrying about me."

Alec was so understanding, and always ready to help. He finished with a kiss on my forehead. "With Jack's love," he added, and went back to reassure Jack.

Next morning I was at the hostel, thanks to reliable Trevor. I found Jack still in bed, though none the worse for his experience. I learned that he had suffered "something with a very long name which induced rapid heart-beat!" No treatment was prescribed by the consultant. Jack was convinced that his heart had stopped beating, at the time. He had also been told that it could happen again, though not necessarily so.

It seemed as though we were being reminded of our own vulnerability, but these unpleasant incidents, we feel, also helped to cement our relationship.

12: Just Daydreams

Life was to leave us undisturbed for a time, though perhaps a little reflective and subdued. For me, another friendship had been developing, which would be more significant than I first realised. It came through my indirect contacts with the Muscular Dystrophy Group, whose local branch had started in 1960. A publicity film was shown at a Young Wives' Group, when it was generally requested that anyone with a car and a little time to spare "might consider taking a sufferer out for a ride". Mildred, then in her late twenties, offered her services.

Shortly afterwards her husband, Bill, called to see me. He explained that my name had been suggested because I lived nearest to his family. He was serious and gentle, and cautiously asked if I would like to go out with them one Sunday afternoon.

I had, of course, met several "do-gooders", and I would be the last person to use that term derisively. On the other hand, I was wary of rash offers which, although made with sincerity at the time, could often lead to disappointment.

However, Bill seemed the reliable kind, even on that first meeting. I readily agreed. My Sundays, like any other day, were usually spent in bed, and the prospect of being driven to some pretty spot, wherever it was, appealed to me enormously. Being in different company was also a promising proposition.

Thus, my new friendship began. Mildred and Bill took me for a couple of trips to the coast, and then I was invited to tea. In and out of the car, Bill lifted me well. Never once did I feel a burden. I was accepted on equal terms and I appreciated it.

In their home I found pleasure with their children, their records and their books. They generously shared a part of their life with me, in a way which I shall always remember.

Although life had afforded Mildred and Bill a far better education than I had, I still appreciated our conversations, which opened my mind to many new interests. Mildred was a trained teacher, though with her children, four-years-old Andrew and Sarah only eighteen months, she was not working then. As a Probation Officer, Bill was slowly climbing the promotion ladder.

Within a year, however, Bill was transferred to County Durham, and the family had to move. I naturally missed them, but we kept in touch by post, and before long, they invited me for a holiday. I was reluctant to leave Jack, but he insisted that I should go. Mildred and Bill had always listened interestedly whenever I talked about Jack, so they were sure to let me telephone him. They appeared to understand the deadlock situation which Jack and I had almost happily settled into. Indeed, we had "almost happily accepted it"—but not quite!

Mildred and Bill seemed gifted at treating me as normal. They almost convinced me that I was not disabled. My confidence was growing.

Jack once wrote, "It often happens, while following the contours of Life's bumpy road, that one reaches new peaks from which to survey the scene below. One is presented with a different aspect, and is therefore able to see a situation from a new angle. . . ."

I suspect that this was beginning to happen to me.

It was this new thought process which seemed to lead Jack and me into excited conversations on the practicalities of living together. It became a frequent topic, as we would discuss in detail the arrangements necessary in our "dream home", covering everything from the kitchen lay-out to the basic structure of the dwelling. We revelled in exploring every possibility of making money, which seemed to be the biggest, if not the only, stumbling block between us and the realisation of our ambitions.

"If only I had a job," Jack would sigh, "at least we could save more, and have a go at it all."

I used to agree, but would often reach an optimistic conclusion. "Perhaps you'll win on the Premium Bonds one day, you know?"

We fully realised that we were only day-dreaming. The one visible symbol of the bonds between us was the Eternity Ring which I wore on my wedding finger. To the outside world, this affinity was the total extent of our mutual commitment. But who could blame people for such short-sightedness? After all, we never revealed our hopes or desires to anyone. And few could have realised the true depths of our feelings.

But we bore no grudges. Fate may have been unkind in presenting us with these limitations, but she had restored the balance with this gift of pure love and companionship which could not be repressed. The big question was—how to use that gift?

13: Shall We Get Married?

Nineteen-sixty-six began excitedly. Trevor and Freda were expecting their first baby in July. I was to have two weeks' holiday with Mildred and Bill in March. Jack and I were becoming accustomed to sharing the joys of others, and were grateful for their involvement. Life seemed good all round.

Even so, we were completely innocent of the fact that this year would be of great personal importance to us.

My own family life was just as interesting. Michael and David were both married, and Gerard was attending a Catholic Junior School. Two extra members of the household were Eileen and Joey, whom Mum had fostered from the ages of five and three respectively. The house was always a hive of activity after school, with homework, piano lessons, dancing, cub scouts. I happily shared in the children's excitement, and tried sympathetically to sort out their little problems whenever necessary. I enjoyed it all, really.

My mother was well, mercifully, but my father still attended to most of my needs. We had changed our vehicle for a third time, and now had an ex-ambulance Bedford. There had been no harmonica trips since Sheila died, but we all went out together occasionally, and Jack would often spend a Sunday at home with us. Eleven years had passed since we first met.

We went to Gorleston Holiday Camp as usual in September. We eagerly anticipated our whole week of togetherness, though bracing ourselves for the inevitable painful parting at the end of it. For me, being with Jack quite simply completed my entire world. Everything seemed then to fall into its rightful place. Jack admitted to enjoying the same secure comforting feelings. But we still reconciled ourselves at this level.

We now knew all the secluded spots in the camp which were accessible by wheelchair! We were familiar with the routine, and planned our days accordingly. But there were no midnight jaunts for us now. Our health was fairly good at this time, and we saw the wisdom in doing our best to keep it that way.

Certainly, at the start of this particular holiday there was no inkling of the plans we were to embark on. But a trivial incident seemed to ignite us into action.

Alex, a disabled friend whom we met only annually, came upon us one sunny afternoon as we sat in our now familiar close position.

"Hello, you two. You know, it's very embarrassing. Hardly dare turn a corner," he said in his amusing Yorkshire accent. "When are you getting married?"

We joked back, "When we can afford it."

"Only costs 7/6d. for a licence," came the cheeky rejoinder.

Alex, several years our senior, was happily married to a nursing sister. His dependency on a wheelchair had not deterred him from living life to the full. His philosophy tended to be sound, and many were enlightened by his little words of wisdom. His latest remark was to have a big influence on us.

We sat by the swimming pool until the air turned chilly. Most people, we guessed, were changing in readiness for the evening meal. We were alone. We watched a thousand reflections dancing on the blue water, as the sun sank in the sky.

"Why don't we get married, Jack?"

There was silence for a moment. Jack never answers quickly at any time! He stroked my hand thoughtfully. "Yes, well, I suppose there's nothing to stop us doing that much."

Again there was silence. Then I suddenly realised the seriousness of my question.

"Whatever will our parents say?"

"What will everyone else say?" Jack added.

"I don't care what other people think," I said with more conviction, "It would just be nice to have our relationship recognised, don't you think?"

Jack's eyes looked dreamy, as he said: "Well, at least we could sleep together when on holiday!"

It was as simple as that. There was no romantic proposal. We were well aware of our mutual feelings. It seemed a small step to take, with little drama attached. After all, we were only planning a wedding ceremony—not a lifetime together. Much as we would have liked to do the whole thing properly, it seemed beyond our comprehension.

For the rest of that week, we discussed our new and exciting idea at every opportunity. With my Catholic background we knew it had to be a Church wedding. But it would just be a small affair, with our families and close friends. My mother must be the first to know, and I planned how to break the news, whilst reassuring her that she would not be financially implicated in the arrangements. It all seemed straightforward, and our confidence was sent soaring. I liked the light of anticipation in Jack's eyes as they met mine across the table, or during the evening get-togethers. I could not wait to make my important declaration as soon as I got home. Then we would be free to inform everyone else.

But once home, my courage left me! Without Jack's presence, the strength of my own conviction deserted me completely. Suddenly, I thought how ridiculous it would all appear. We would be the talk of the neighbourhood. Other handicapped couples had become engaged before, only to be treated with amused sympathy.

"Well, if they like to pretend, there's no harm in it, really."

How could I now explain the depth and sincerity of our feelings? How could I possibly describe the meaning behind our decision? So far, we had escaped the need for any such explanation, but now we would be leaving ourselves open to the same patronising comments. I searched for reasons to quell the expected avalanche of criticism.

Visiting Jack later that week, I shamefully admitted my sudden loss of nerve when it came to telling my mother about our wedding plans. He was as understanding as always. On reflection, we then decided that a big announcement was not appropriate. Instead, we would proceed in a somewhat more discreet manner.

"Let's become engaged first, and name the day later on," suggested Jack. "This will allow time for people to get accustomed to the new situation. I can buy you an engagement ring for Christmas."

I readily concurred.

We decided to purchase the ring through a mail-order firm, to save getting ourselves involved in shopping expeditions which could not be as private as we wanted. I chose a fairly inexpensive ring which had a single zircon set in a white gold band. It was beautiful to me.

With each week approaching Christmas, I braced myself to speak to Mother, but courage always failed me at the last minute. Time was running out. I simply had to get the news out soon. I was not going back on my word, that was for certain.

Then one day, it slipped out so easily that I wondered what all my fears were for.

"Guess what Jack's buying me for Christmas, Mum?"

There was a pause while she pondered.

"An engagement ring," I said softly, to conceal any embarrassment.

"Oh, that's nice," Mother replied, almost blankly.

I knew that this was not enough, and I wanted her to grasp the full implication. Taking a deep breath, I persisted. "I do mean an engagement ring, Mum. It's a promise to marry, you know. We hope to arrange it for next year."

She still seemed unperturbed, saying, "Well, you know what you want to do."

The truth was out. There were no questions and no ridicule. But this was only the beginning. The relief had an intoxicating effect on me. I prattled on whilst the going was good, assuring Mother that no expense would be incurred for her or Dad. The wedding would not appear to make any difference to anyone else, but as I told her, it was important to Jack and me. To my complete surprise, Mum seemed quite placid about the whole thing.

Jack would be pleased that my mother was now in possession of the facts as they stood, anyway. He had already resolved to write to my parents, if I could not bring myself to tell them!

When hearing the news, many people failed completely to understand.

"Didn't realise you felt that way about each other."

"What's the point?" said others. "How will you feel married?"

We only smiled away such reactions, even though we felt hurt.

Nevertheless, we did have our supporters. Trevor and Freda were pleased for us, and offered all their help. "About time, too," said Alec simply, though it spoke volumes for him. Mildred and Bill remarked that they wondered why we had not done it before. That, too, was a warm response.

Already we felt united. We could take all the queries. The decision to marry, without any obvious changes in our circumstances, would appear futile. We appreciated that. But nothing would deter us now. Our minds were made up.

Gradually, as the news spread everyone got used to the fact that Jack and Margaret were getting married. Furthermore the date had been fixed for Saturday July 8th 1967, to coincide with Jack's birthday.

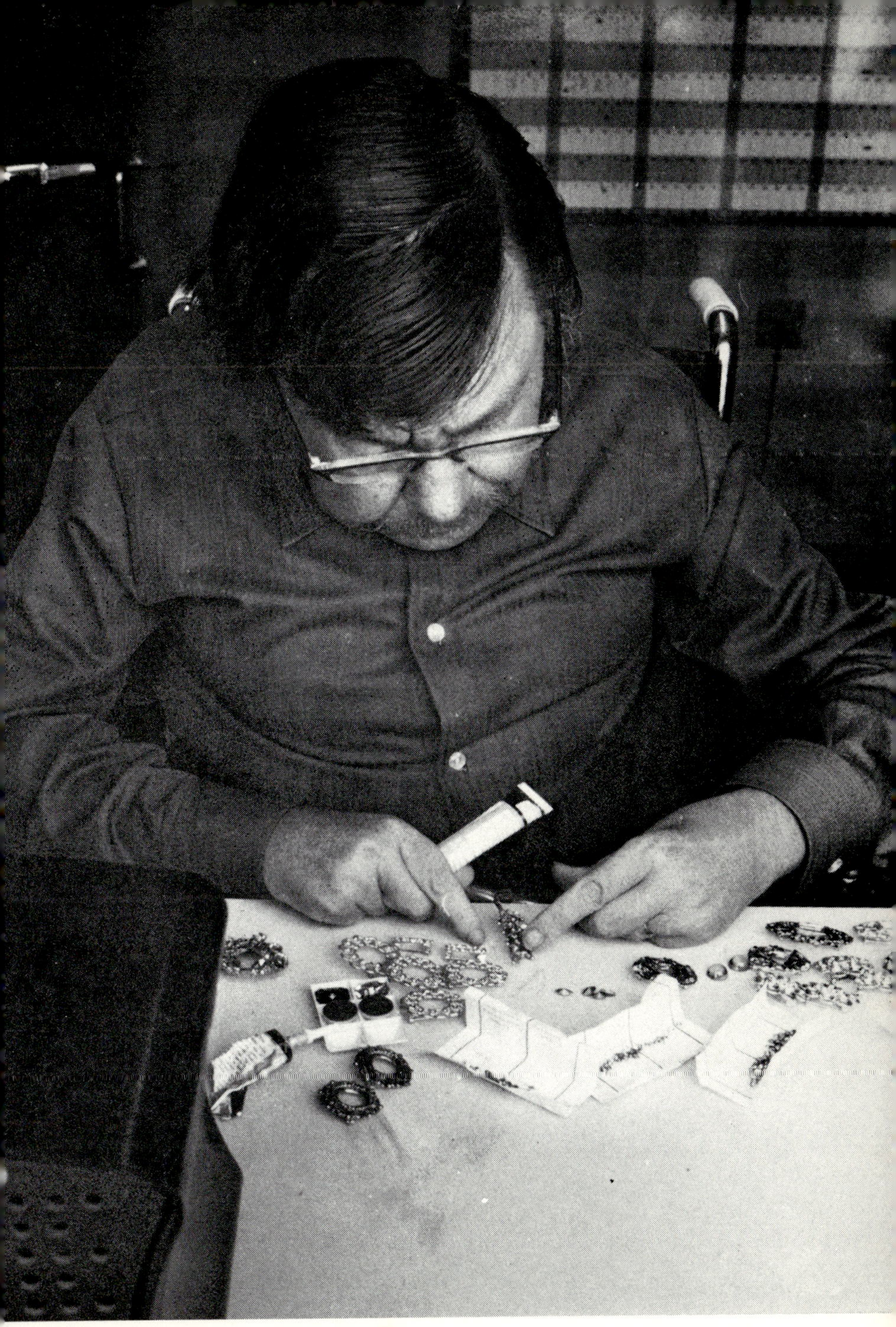

Jack's new venture was assembling costume jewellery.

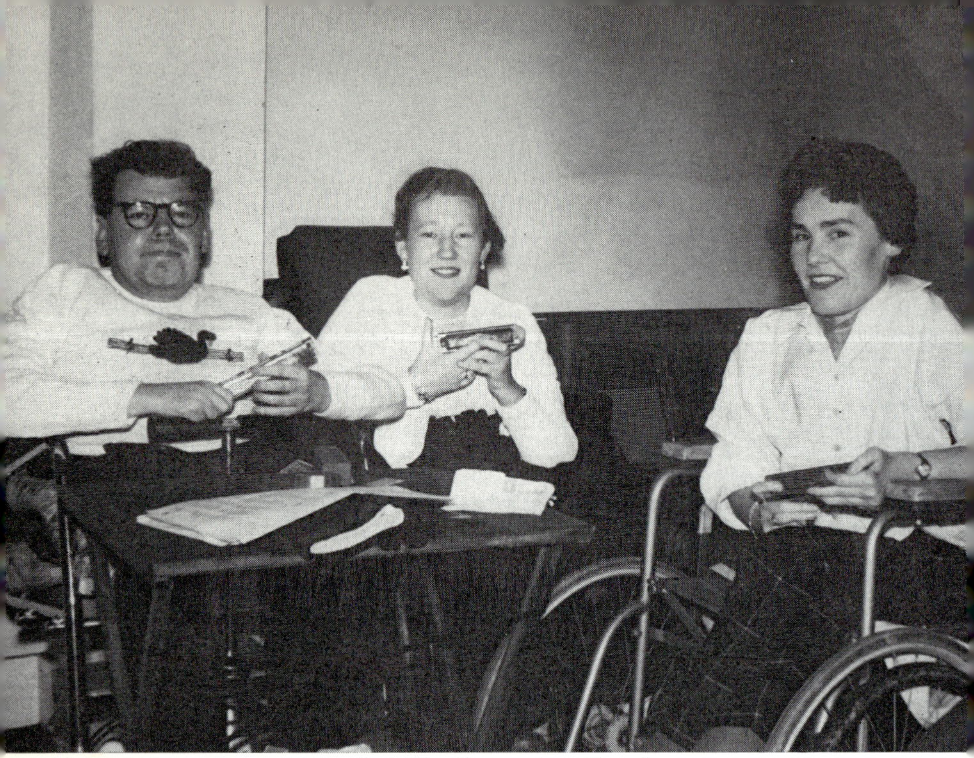

Thus, we formed our group called 'The Harmonicas Three'...

By the swimming pool at Gorleston Camp, 1964.

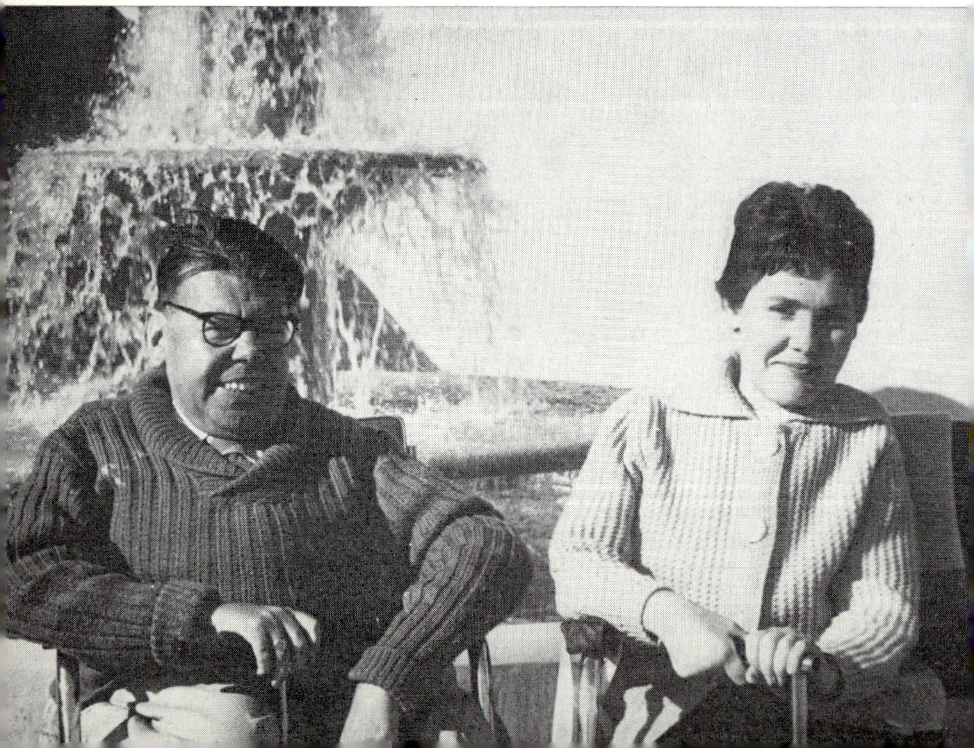

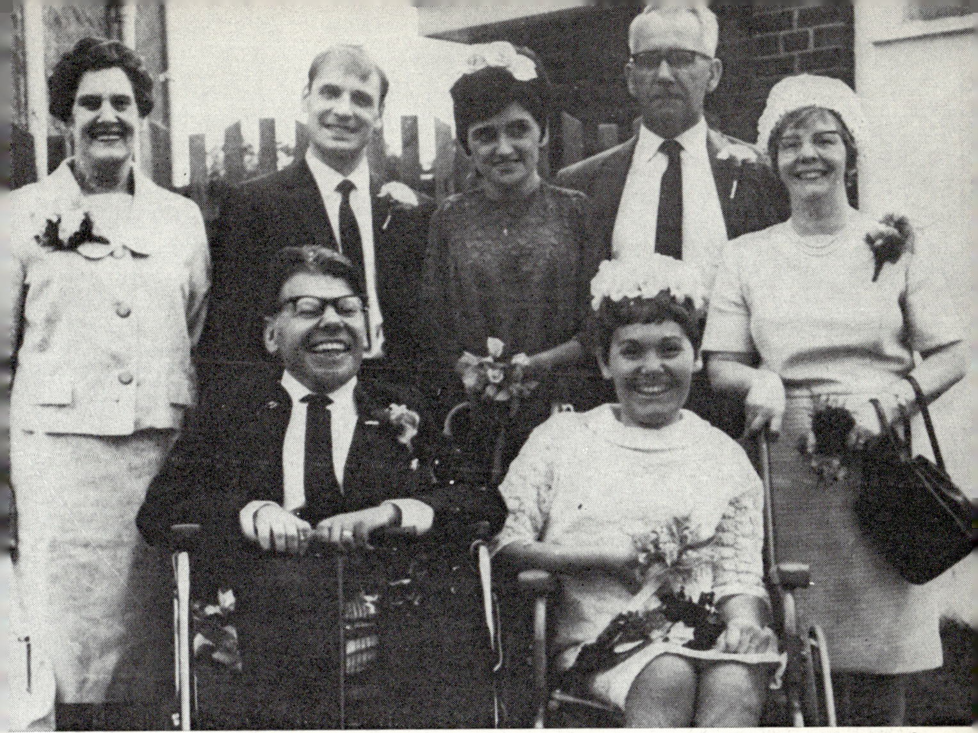

The Wedding – standing (left to right): Jack's mother; Trevor and Freda; Margaret's father and mother.

Our great day arrived . . .

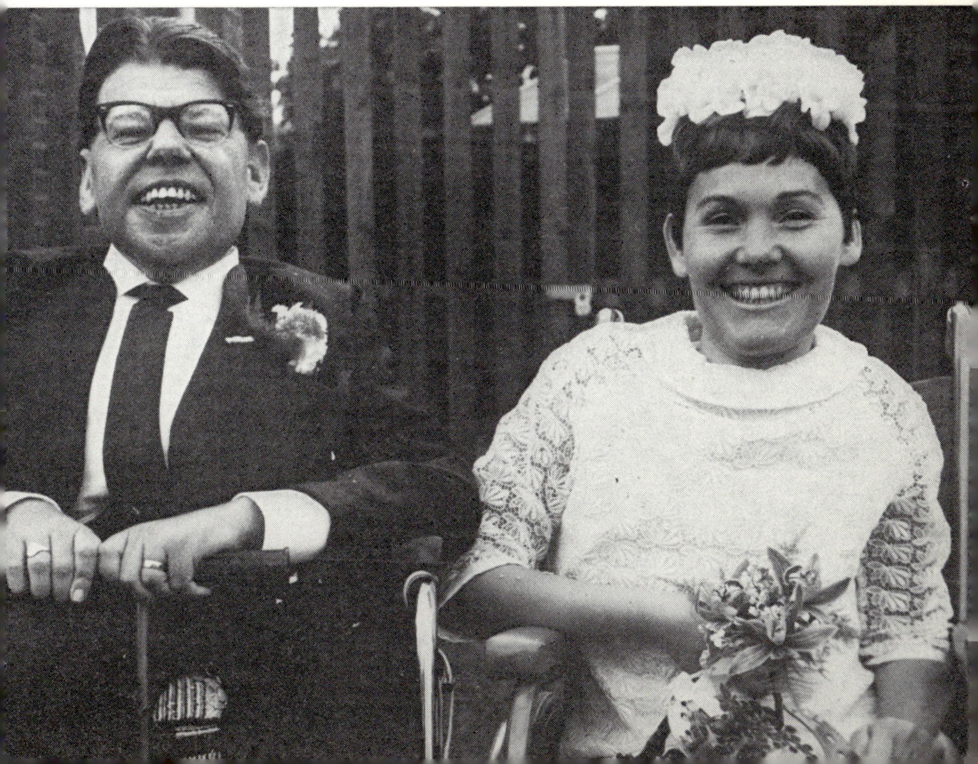

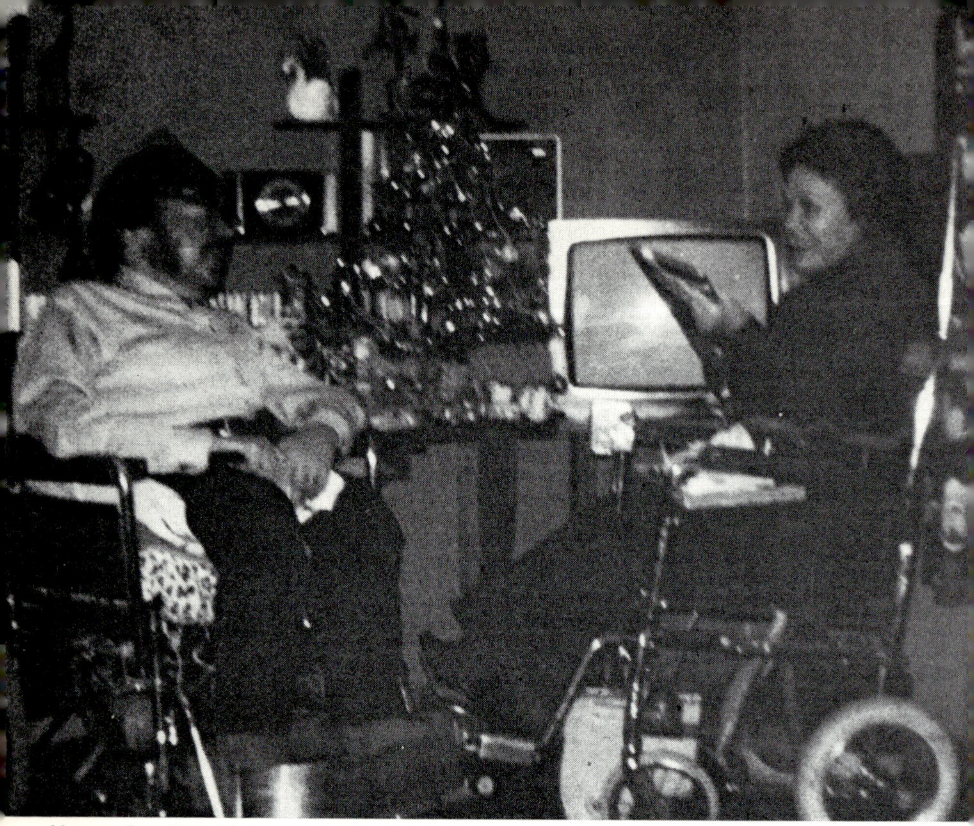

Above: Our first Christmas in the flat (1969).

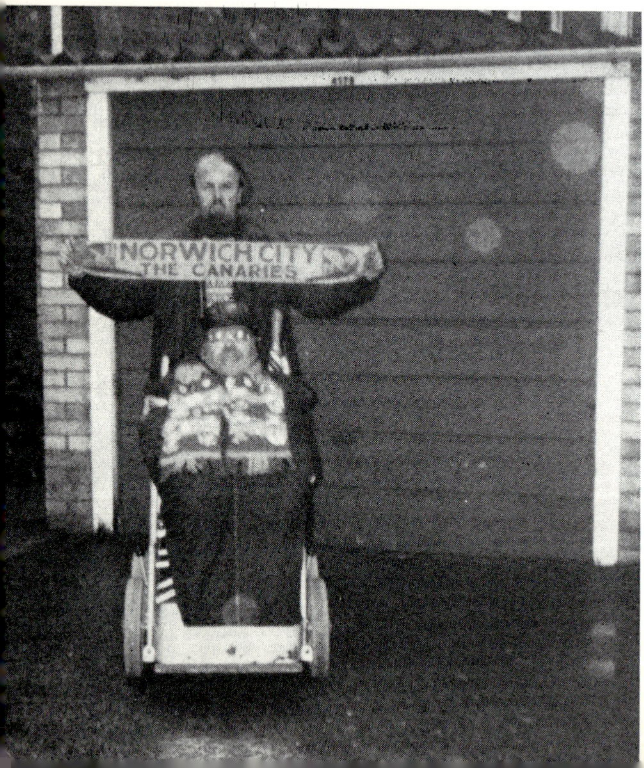

Left: Come on, Norwic
Jack and his friend Mi
prepare for the footba
match.

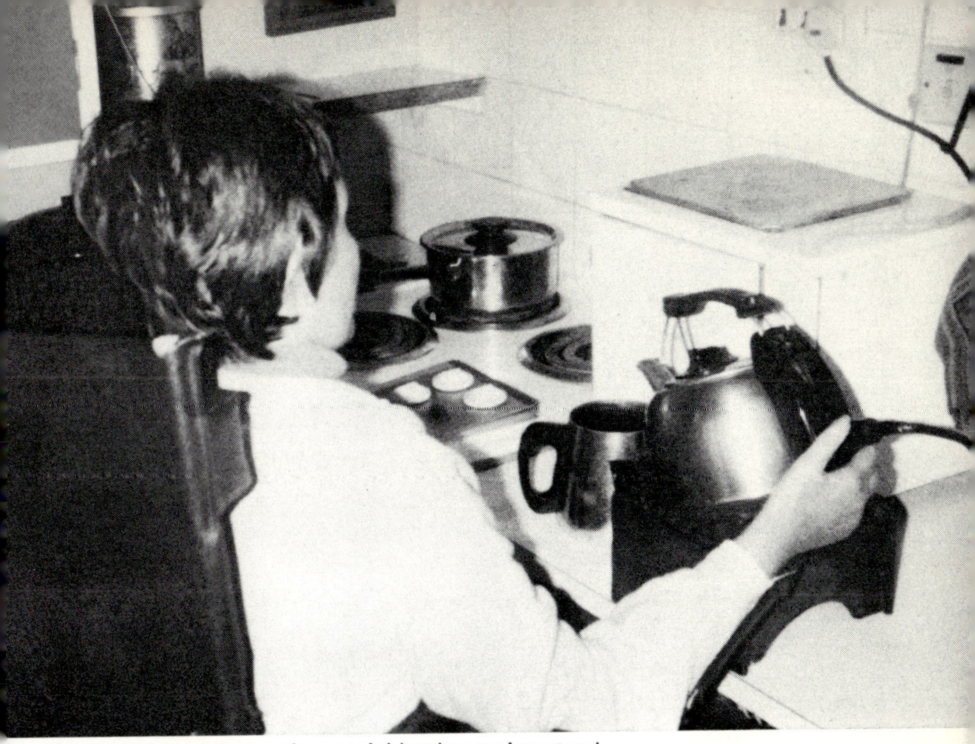

Margaret demonstrates the special kettle pouring stand.

Margaret gets down to the washing up.

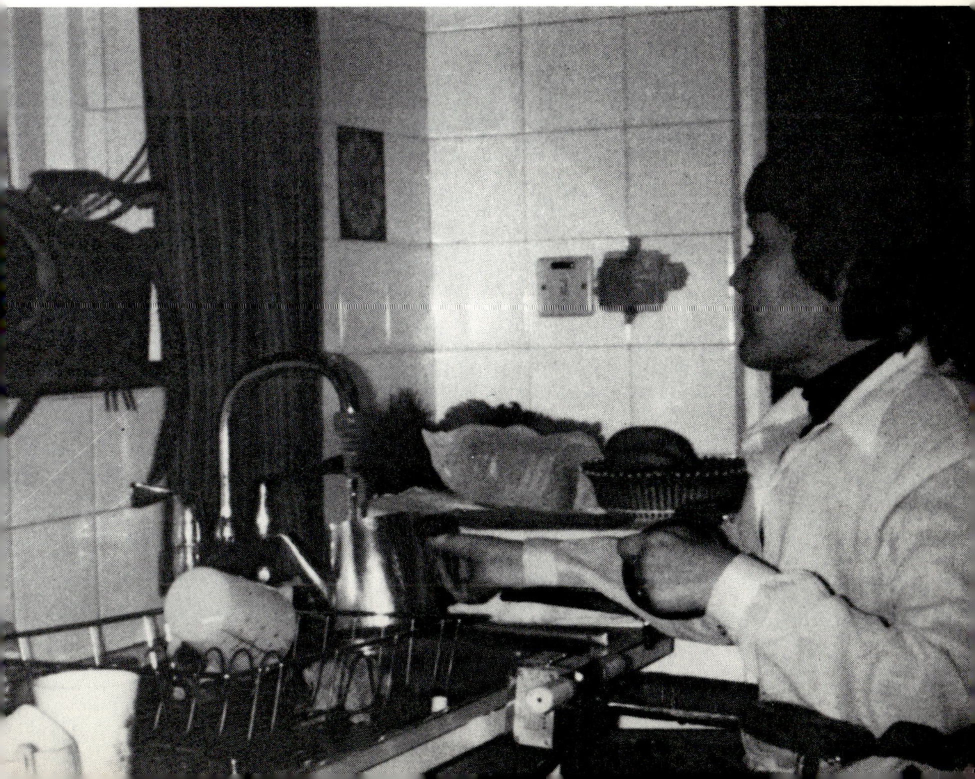

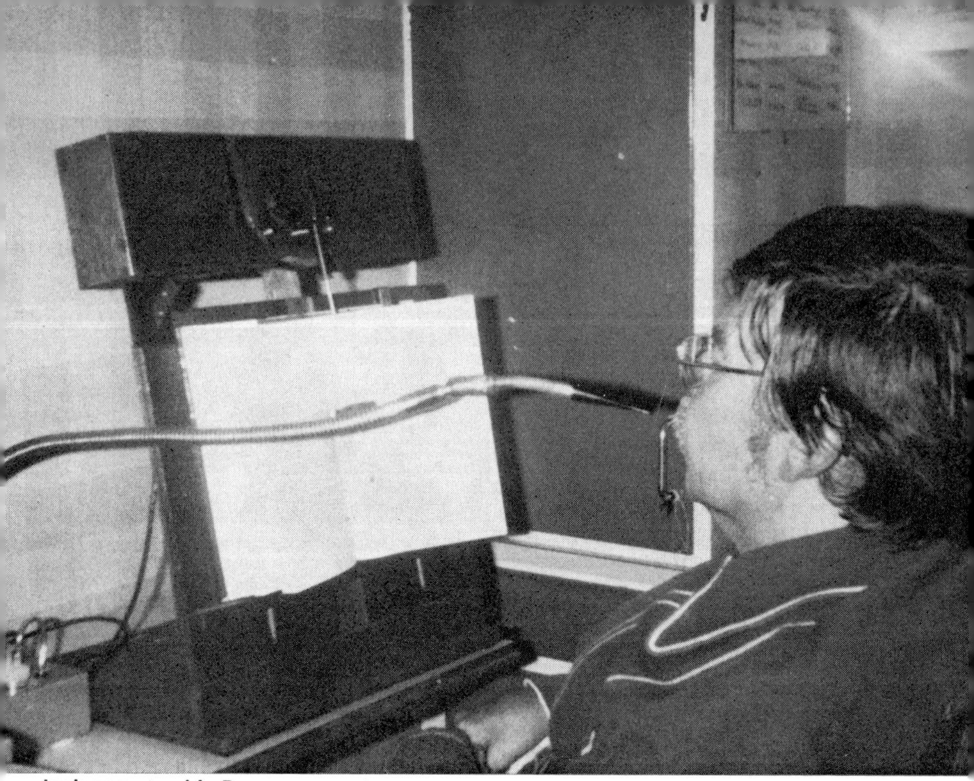

Jack operates his Possum page turner.

Jack types by holding a short stick in both hands.

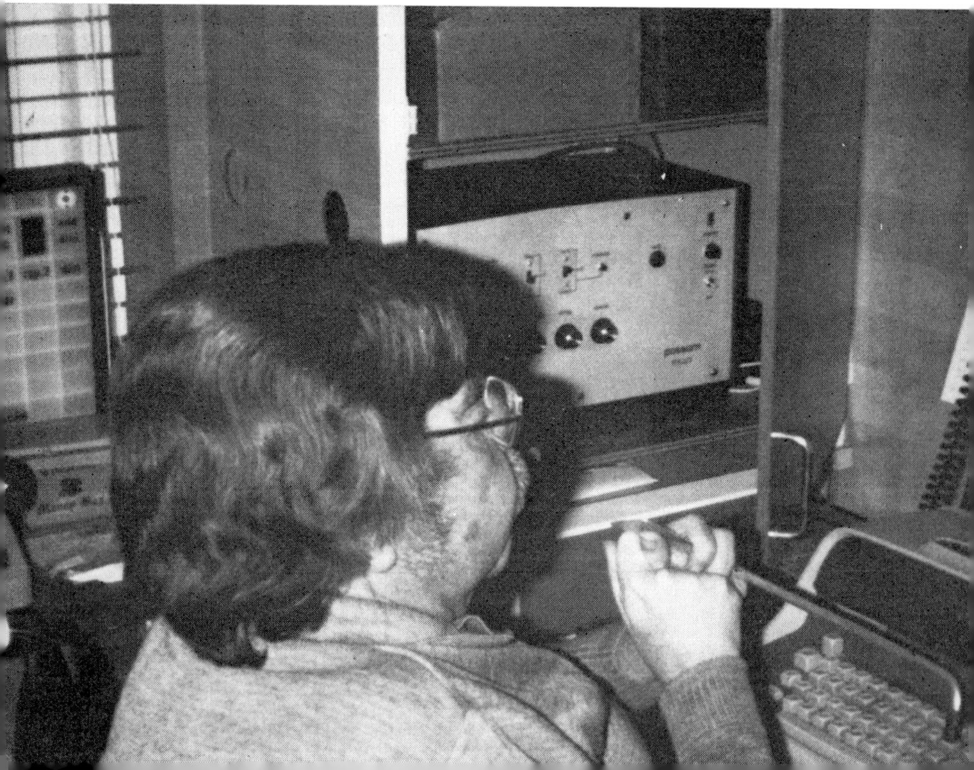

Right: Margaret and Gerry sort the toys before a Toy Library session

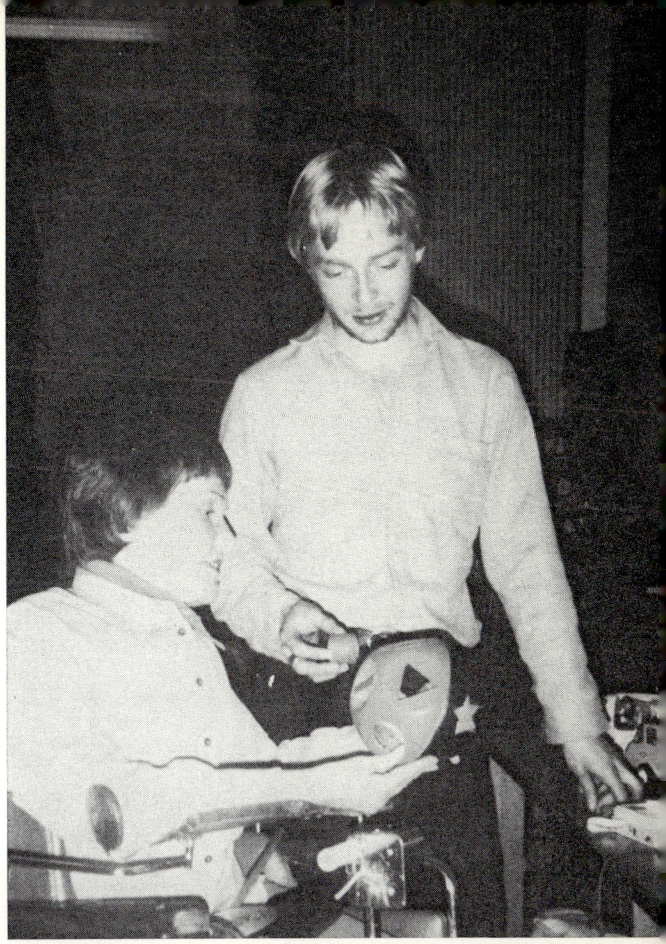

Below: Gerry and Margaret check the files on Toy Library members.

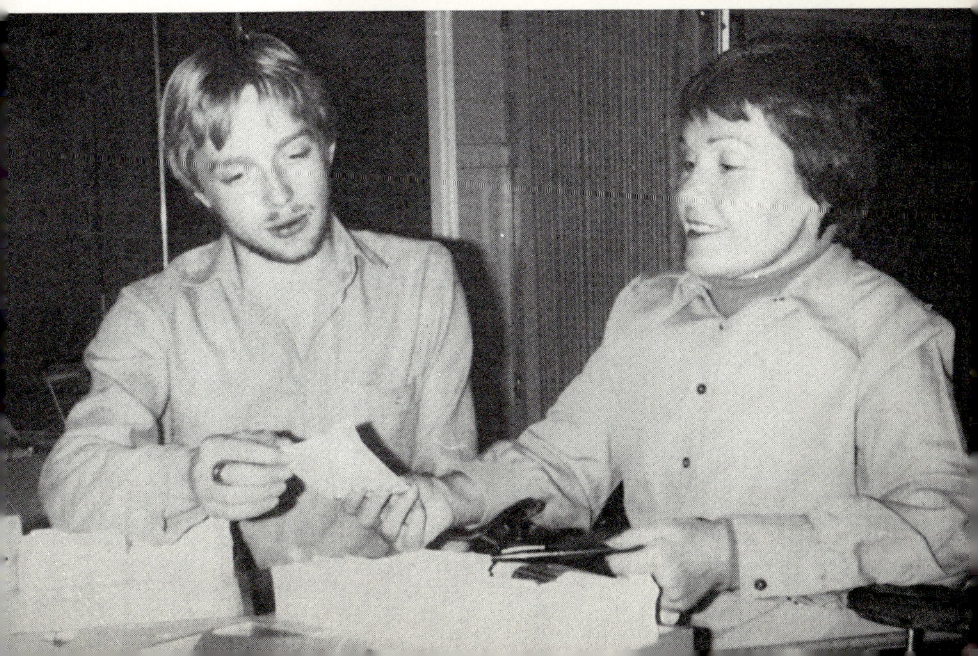

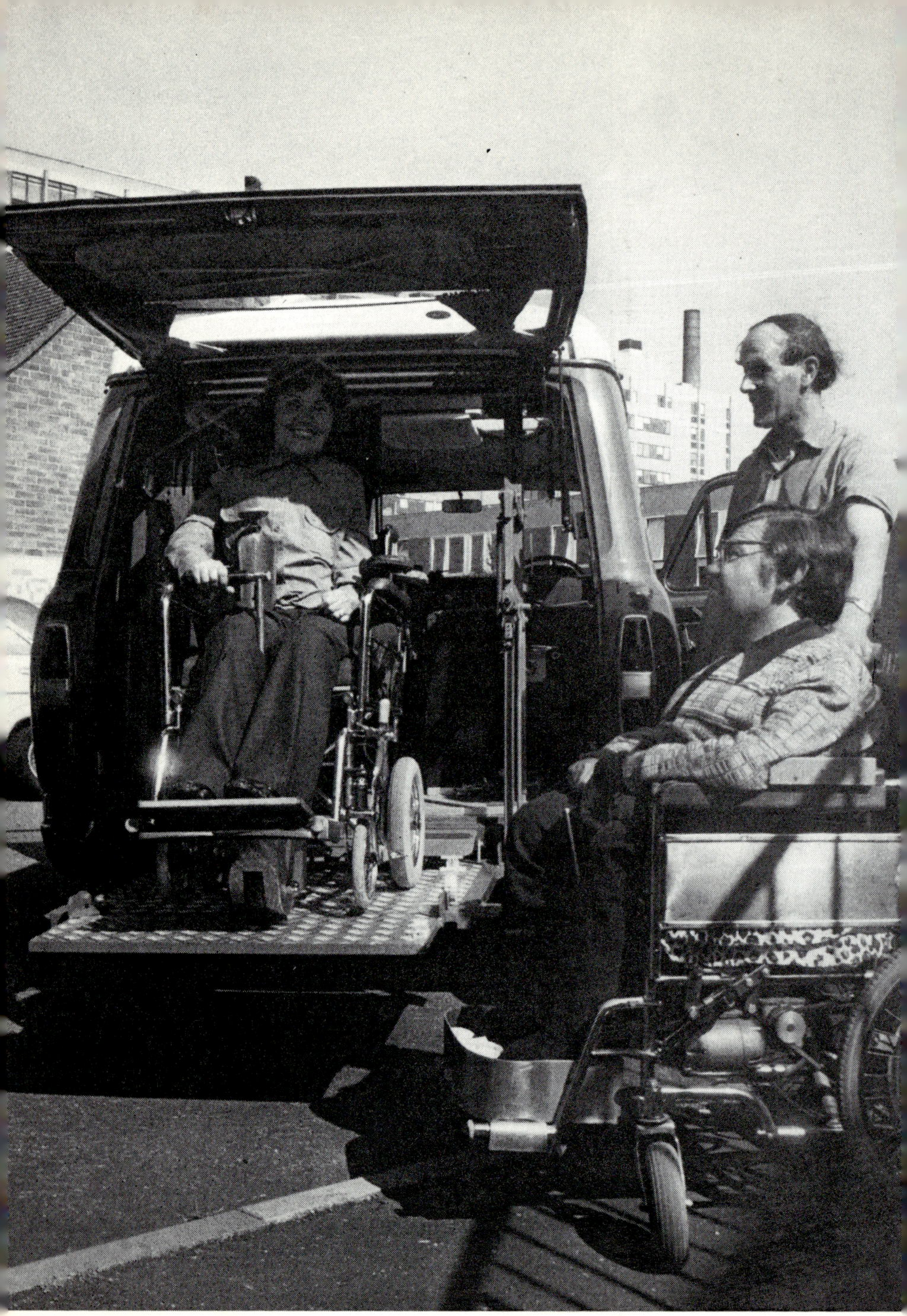

We took delivery of a smart, red dormobile.

14: Wedding Plans

The months leading up to our wedding were busy. We made the necessary arrangements with the local Parish priest and the registrar, and hoped to make it a quiet affair with just our families present. Then a few friends were carefully selected. Gradually the numbers crept to seventy guests, and we had to arrange a buffet reception in the adjoining church hall! Freda was happy to be my Maid of Honour, and Trevor to be Best Man.

Choosing our wedding rings was a bit more complicated. Going out together would have involved two others again, and those precious intimate moments would be lost. So we asked a voluntary shopper for the hostel's residents to request a small selection on approval from the jewellers. It was a bold request indeed, but the lady was entrusted with three men's and three ladies' rings! We tried them on in the quiet seclusion of Jack's room. I chose a patterned white gold band, to match my engagement and eternity rings, while Jack's ring was faceted in yellow gold.

Keeping costs to the minimum, I decided to make my own wedding outfit. It was a simple white lace two-piece, lined with satin. I later matched this with a small floral coronet, and shoes, whilst on a rare shopping expedition with Freda and Trevor. I also made Freda's short turquoise dress.

But what would Jack wear for the occasion? He never had the courage to be measured for a suit, believing it impossible to fit his awkward shape smartly. However, he did let me try making him a jacket, and bought some charcoal-grey material to match his ready-made trousers. He seemed confident that my efforts would make him presentable enough. Looking back,

E

that seems strange now, when he thinks nothing of entering the local shop for a tailor-made suit or coat.

In traditional style, Jack and Trevor celebrated with their own little Stag Party, settling in a pub where they enjoyed the music. Meantime, Freda and I were left preparing some trifle for the buffet. Her small kitchen suited me fairly well for working. I had arranged to stay the night at their house, so that Trevor could take me to the hairdresser next morning.

A beaming Trevor eventually returned home, obviously and happily tiddly, and pleased to inform us that Jack was in a similar state when he left him. Whereupon Trevor bumped into the table, and all the trifle cases turned upside down on the floor! Freda and I were flabbergasted. We did not know whether to laugh or cry.

"Oh, Trevor. You clumsy clot!" we shouted in unison.

During all these plans, one day at the hostel, I met Miss Elizabeth Barnes. She expressed keen interest in the news, which was now spreading fast. I can still recall her gentle expression as she enquired: "And you intend to live as you are now, even after the wedding?"

I nodded, adding, "Unless we can find a place where disabled couples can live together."

My comments were merely by the way, since I was then unaware of Miss Barnes' influential position as Assistant Chief Welfare Officer.

"We'd also like a honeymoon together, but don't really know of anywhere to go."

Miss Barnes' tall, neat figure bent low, as she said quietly and with great understanding, "I'll make a few enquiries."

We were soon to learn about a WRVS Centre in Surrey. It would be our very first holiday without friends who understood our needs completely. But carried along by my enthusiasm, Jack seemed ready for anything! Fifty pounds for a fortnight's stay seemed an absolute fortune to us. But before we could start worrying about it, the local branch of the Muscular

Dystrophy Group had offered us a grant. It seemed too good to be true.

We were not expecting to have a home of our own, and so wedding presents were unnecessary. Nevertheless, many people insisted on giving us cash. There were some very touching responses, too. A cheque from Mildred and Bill had an accompanying note simply saying "To buy a little time together."

15: The Honeymoon

Our great day arrived! When I awoke, it was a grey, wet day, but I cared little for the weather. It was our happy day. After I had visited the hairdresser, Trevor, Freda and I proceeded to my home to change into our finery.

Meanwhile, at the hostel the Staff were buzzing round Jack. They enjoyed getting him smartly dressed, though there was a good deal of ribbing and hilarity in the process. Alec and his wife, Laura, would be taking him to the church in their suitably large van, and then return for me at home.

By 1.30 p.m. my mother was down at the church, excitedly distributing the carnation buttonholes. Jack duly arrived there, pleased to see everyone, but mainly Trevor and Freda.

Only Dad and I were left at home, awaiting our transport. It was a suspended moment of anticipation and nervousness. My father, non-committal as always, said little. I sat ready in my wheelchair, clutching my spray of three orchids. Hair immaculate, make-up complete, left me nothing to fiddle with. I tried to calm myself. But the enormity of the situation had hit me at last. The house was silent, and I was scared.

Alec greeted me with a kiss on the forehead, took my chair, and we were on our way. His Bedford Workobus gleamed from meticulous polishing, and was decorated with white carnations and ribbons. I could feel the neighbours watching as my chair mounted the wooden ramp into the vehicle. But I could not return their gaze.

The church was but a short ride away. The Press report stated "The bride arrived five minutes early." Dad clasped the handles of my chair, and soon we were moving slowly down the aisle, to the usual Wedding March. I wanted *The Arrival of the Queen of Sheba*, but the organist could not play it!

Numerous clichés flashed through my mind as we progressed down the aisle, more slowly than usual, to keep pace with Freda's tiny steps. All the time, I could not believe it was happening.

At last I reached Jack's side at the altar. Breaking tradition, I sat on his right-hand side, for an easier exchange of rings. He looked so alive and happy, and smart in every detail. We glanced at each other almost mischievously. My broad wink showed him that all was well with me, though it was hardly the greeting he expected! My brother Gerard, now eleven years old, served as the Altar Boy. It was all real after all, and happening to us. The Service was simple, and full of true meaning.

There must have been mixed feelings amongst those in the congregation. Miss Barnes summed up her own impressions later, in a spontaneously worded letter which said: "It finally confirmed all I had believed so far."

Little did we realise what a big influence she would have on our future.

Outside the church once more, the sun began to penetrate the clouds in time for the photographs. There were jocular remarks about the numbers of children clustered around the bride and groom! Sitting on my lap was one-year-old Andrew, son of Trevor and Freda.

"About time you got married, isn't it?," jibed someone.

Then we joined the party in the crowded reception room, and thereafter time passed quickly. Before long I was changed into my self-styled lilac going-away suit, and Jack was making his little speeches.

We boarded the Bedford, and departed at 3.30 p.m. A long journey lay ahead to our honeymoon destination, and Alec and Laura had arranged to stay overnight with some friends in Surrey. The sun shone brilliantly as we set off. Bright conversation accompanied the first part of the journey. Then there were different feelings coming over us. We were travelling into the unknown.

Many uncertainties crowded our minds during those four hours on the road. What kind of treatment would we get? So much depended on how Jack was seated in his chair, for sometimes he could not feed himself. Would there be any expert hands available at all? We became less and less talkative, but fortunately Alec and Laura seemed unaware.

Finally we turned off the narrow country road and into the bumpy driveway. We parked outside the lovely old house, and immediately liked what we saw of the trees, lawns and flower-beds. Alec went inside to deal with the formalities, and we were warmly received in a large room with a beautiful view.

"Supper is over, I'm afraid, but would you like a cup of tea?"

We had resolved to guard our secret of being newly-weds as far as possible. Therefore, we hoped it surprised everyone when the removal of Jack's coat showered confetti over the floor!

"Oh, we've been to a wedding today," we excused ourselves.

We drank our tea, and Alec and Laura left, giving a telephone number for any necessary contact.

Our bedroom was spacious and inviting, and the flower arrangements made it homely. My own spray of orchids was put in water.

"The bride gave me her bouquet," I bluffed again. These weak attemps at hiding the facts amused me, though we must have been as obvious as if we had hung a "Just Married" notice around our necks.

With the unpacking completed, we were left alone to take stock of our new surroundings. Room 14 seemed very pleasant indeed. The large patio doors overlooked another lawn fringed with rose bushes, and a huge oak tree shaded the paved area immediately outside. Only one thing spoilt the illusion. The two hospital-type beds were meaningfully separated by the bedside lockers! Well, perhaps our hosts could be excused this once. After all, they were not supposed to know that Mr and Mrs Wymer were newly married.

Having been used always to being told what to do, we were soon surprised to find that we ourselves had to call the tune. Guests could stay up as late as they liked, but by 9.30 p.m. we were both feeling very tired. Jack elected to be first, and set off to find a helper. It took some courage in a strange place, feeling exhausted as he was from the day's exceptional circumstances. But the bed-time routine was made easier by the ready willingness of the two young men he chose. Not only was he made comfortable, but he succeeded in getting the beds pushed together.

I allowed Jack half an hour, then I approached our room, when the helpers were just folding his clothes. Jack was lying down, looking relaxed and happy. There was an air of light-hearted amusement.

"Your husband's a right comedian," said one.

"Your Husband." I considered the phrase briefly. It impressed me. It was the first time anyone had said it. I smiled then, not so much from hearing the phrase, but more from relief. Jack must be feeling good, for his sense of humour to show already!

The lads continued joking with my two girls. Now all fears were banished. The atmosphere was warm and bright, and these young people were out to please us. Thoughts of embarrassment were ignored. It mattered little who we were, or what we could do.

I was soon undressed and settled down. Our young friends were happy to respond to every request, and we were determined to get as close as our unco-operative bodies permitted. When it came to moving me near to Jack, they got on to the bed as well, and lifted me across, amidst giggles at their own antics!

The trained night-nurse popped in to see that all was well, and having placed the nurse-call bell on its lead for our convenience, all the helpers left the room. At last we were alone.

Snuggled close together, we shared one set of bed-clothes. The warmth we experienced from simply holding hands all those years ago was magnified a million times, and flooded over us. The bed smelled fresh and clean and strange, but Jack smelled just like Jack. So close were our bodies that we could feel and hear our hearts beating in rapid rhythm. For a long time we revelled in these simple sensations. What more could we want? Perhaps our words were those of all young lovers, repeated thousands of times through all ages. Yet they were spoken with a fresh and meaningful importance. Even more important to us was the fact that, despite all the odds, we were now husband and wife. Slowly, gratefully, we fell asleep.

The next day dawned bright with sunshine. In fact, the sun shone brilliantly every day for those two weeks, and we spent much of our time outside, often selecting a quiet corner of the gardens to be left alone together. We felt at peace with the world, and even more in love. We could not get enough of one another.

"I just want all of you, all of the time," Jack once said.

I shared his longing. Just being together seemed such a little to ask.

"Perhaps we'll find out about a suitable place where they accept married couples?" I ventured.

"Attitudes will have to change a lot before that happens." Jack was less optimistic.

"Never mind. We'll be together one day, I'm sure."

There the matter would rest, as our attention was caught by the sudden appearance of two squirrels playing "statues" on the lawn.

We soon became friendly with our fellow guests and helpers, and often shared a jig-saw or a hand at cards. Outings were arranged, but we preferred to stay put. There was the inevitable chess set with which to amuse ourselves, or the radio and books. We sat watching the Test Match on television for several hours, punctuated with trying to solve crossword puzzles.

"Who'd have thought honeymoons were made of this?" quipped Jack one day.

On the last night, we lay awake for hours, clinging to all those treasured memories. But we were determined to be together somehow, even if it meant leaving our home town to find suitable accommodation. Meantime, we consoled ourselves with the thought that there would be other holidays. And of course Trevor's and Freda's offers to stay remained open.

Almost regretfully, Alec and Laura arrived punctually on the Saturday morning. Significantly, the sun had gone. The return journey was dull. Silently, we each prepared ourselves for yet another inevitable separation.

But we would be eased into the reality this time, by a further three days' stay with our friends. So when we unloaded at the hostel, we waited for Trevor to fetch us in his car. In this way, we were gradually brought down to earth, and things turned out quite well for that.

16: Can Dreams Come True?

Back in the old routine once more, little had changed on the surface. One subtle difference, however, was that the front of my Supplementary Benefit Order Book now carried my married name.

Three weeks after returning from honeymoon, my usual Tuesday letter from Jack contained news which was almost unbelievable. His Social Worker had had a confidential chat with him, and in Jack's own words "had asked if we'd like to live in a flat of our own, and I said 'You give us the chance'. . . ."

That was all the Social Worker would say, except that he would be in touch.

I read the letter over and over again, before I replied. Could this mean that our dreams might come true after all? But so many obstacles had to be overcome, and I dare not become too hopeful. Nevertheless, I reassured Jack that I, for one, would do my utmost to achieve our aim—if we could believe it was possible.

A month went by with no further news. I grew impatient to know whether or not we could have faith in such a project, and decided to write direct to Miss Barnes. Another few days dragged on, until she replied carefully: "I'm sure Jack must have told you that we want to help all we can. But since nothing like this has happened before, we can't make any real promises." We were really putting her on the spot to make decisions which were beyond even her control. Looking back, I am positive that she wanted to see us living happily together —almost as much as we wanted it ourselves. But her letter ended: "What do *you* feel should be the first move?"

Our minds buzzed with ideas, and as a result I told Miss

Barnes of our discovery of an Assessment Centre near Oxford, where there was a "Trial Flat" in which disabled people could practise daily living.

It seemed an ideal place for us to start, and Miss Barnes arranged a meeting to discuss the matter fully. We gathered in Jack's room at the hostel, and she outlined the procedure. Letters of recommendation should be sent to the Centre by our individual doctors. Thereafter, we would be put on the waiting list. It was now September. How long must we wait, we wondered?

In fact, it was March the following year before we could be admitted. A hospital ambulance would collect us, and we would stay at the Centre for two weeks. The ball had started rolling! We were confused as to whether to be pleased or scared. Uncertainties were always a problem. Neither of us felt very fit at the time. Jack still had his irksome bladder trouble, and I just felt generally weary.

We made the long journey together on March 18th, and were eventually shown to the Trial Flat and left to absorb our surroundings. An old drop-leaf table was matched by equally scratched dining chairs, and pushed against the wall. A solid-fuel burner sent its ugly black chimney through the ceiling, while an electric fire stood in the hearth to render it obsolete. A small French door opened on to an enclosed lawn. Under an adjoining window was a Put-U-Up settee. Two odd armchairs, and a chest of drawers completed the assortment of furniture in this part.

Whatever possessed us to come to this? What had we let ourselves in for? Gradually, we began to move around. Jack was used to his powered chair, but my borrowed machine still took some tricky manœuvring. Exploring strange areas was no mean task. A sliding door led us into the kitchen with its conglomeration of utensils and equipment. The sink unit seemed an awkward height for me, and I immediately started wondering how on earth I was going to practise living in such disadvantageous circumstances.

A folding partition separated the "sitting room" from the bedroom, where there were two orthopaedic beds, and the usual lockers. A fearsome-looking hoist dangled ominously on its ceiling track above the beds. We would certainly not be needing that, we thought. Hoists were for big, fat people. My 7½ stone and Jack's 8½ did not warrant such undignified elevation. Where were all these push-button controls? Where was the gleaming equipment, the electronic doors and switches? Obviously, my imagination had run riot. I had much to learn.

Just then, a young nurse called in to put away our belongings, and we were left again with a much needed cup of tea.

Our solitude was short lived. The door opened, and two women introduced themselves respectively as an occupational-therapist and a physiotherapist. Neither title meant much to us, and we were pleased to use their Christian names as offered. They proceeded to take all our particulars in accordance with admitting patients. A less orthodox question, however, was: "Well, now you're here, what do you hope to achieve?"

We hesitantly explained that we hoped to live in our own flat. It still sounded as ridiculous as asking for the moon. Expecting a reaction of hopelessness, we were surprised that the request was met with natural acceptance. Jack mentioned that his powered chair was provided by a charity, and asked if we could both have new ones supplied by the Department of Health and Social Security. They agreed, and I saw "Wheelchair Clinic" written down. So far, so good!

There followed numerous questions about our ability to wash, dress, use the toilet, to which the answers made a string of negatives on the interrogation sheet. That must have sealed our fate once and for all, we thought. No one could do so little and expect so much, surely?

"Do you think we're asking too much?" I ventured.

They smiled reassuringly, saying "We never make promises, but we'll see if various aids might increase your arm movements. At least, you do need new chairs, and so we'll get you mobile."

Asked if they had actually helped any other married couples as helpless as we were to live alone, they shook their heads thoughtfully. "We don't know of any, but there may be more elsewhere."

My heart sank a little lower. Our chances of success seemed remote.

Next morning, we had to stay in bed until the doctor had seen us. Prolonged periods in bed always upset Jack, though it was not so bad for me. But it was to be the worst day we spent there. We did not understand the routine at all, and got very impatient for the doctor's visit. Had we communicated our displeasure to anyone else we would probably have been told in no uncertain terms that there were about twelve other patients suffering the same ordeal. Someone had to be first, and another last.

Finally Doctor Anne appeared, completely disarming us with her heartfelt apologies and delightful personality. She went over us with a medical "fine toothed comb", including simple tests on our muscle power.

Her job was to assess our general health, but we soon discovered that she was equally proficient at giving moral support. All through the blood tests, urine samples, and goodness knows what that followed, Doctor Anne encouraged us, and understood our fears of ridicule. Her sensible and philosophical conclusion was that no marriage could possibly foresee disablement, but at least we knew at the outset what immense problems had to be overcome.

Wheelchair assessments were repeated at intervals during that fortnight, until we each found the type best suited to our needs. We also tried ball-bearing arm supports to assist our arm movements, but here again I came off better than Jack. These arm supports consisted of a metal trough for the arm, pivoting on an elbow-shaped rod, which in turn swivelled in a socket attached to the back of the chair. Early experiments were not very successful, but, determined to prove myself, I managed to use the gadget in my struggles to cook a few dishes, and wash up.

We left the Centre both armed with tablets, for Jack had a urinary bug, and I was slightly anaemic. It was something of an anti-climax. But we would be back, as soon as our new chairs arrived. It could take six months, though, and this seemed an eternity. Meantime, our secret remained with those dedicated to helping us realise our dreams. Others thought we were just having new wheelchairs. Would this be all?

17: Practising for a Future

My weekly visits to the hostel continued. There, Jack and I mulled over our dreams and fears. We still occupied ourselves with our separate handicrafts. I was then making lavender bags for a local firm, which was often hard and exacting work for me. I lived in a continuous muddle of organza material, buckets of lavender, and ribbon bows. Friends approached my bed, jokingly fighting their way through the maze! I was paid one new penny a bag, and worked long hours for £1 a week. But it was satisfying to see the finished hearts, squares and circles all neatly crimped round the edges, and looking shiny and new in their individual cellophane packets.

At least, it was valuable savings to my credit! Social Security Benefit for a person in my position was then £4.50 per week. My extra pound, though hard-earned, was no mean achievement. Jack continued with his jewellery making, but much depended on his own salesmanship and he found that trade was spasmodic. For someone "in care", the pocket money allowance at the time was £1 weekly.

If our private hopes had any substance, we had to think seriously about saving. Were we lucky enough to have a home of our own, we could not expect everything to be laid in our laps. All monies received in lieu of wedding gifts had been put into a joint account, and we planned to add to it. Fortunately, Jack had always been a thrifty person, managing to accumulate a little money in his own way. But I suppose, to be quite honest, we could possibly have mustered no more than £150 between us at that time, and that was hardly sufficient to build a home on, even by our own modest standards.

Nevertheless, we did not allow our low financial backing to disturb us unduly. After all, saving was the one tangible contribution we could make to the future. Everything else, it seemed, was founded on hypotheses. Having set our sights and taken aim, we did not mind how distant the target was. We were content merely to be moving in the right direction.

Six months elapsed quite quickly. Another letter recalling us to the Assessment Centre set our hearts beating excitedly once more. We were ready for anything. We went through all the medical checks again, with gritty determination, and even agreed to experiment with the mechanical hoist! Using a hoist would certainly have its advantages over the expensive and awkward handling of two people. And our daily routines were timed to the minute, in order to try and simulate the real thing.

Having been got up each morning, I would make our cereal breakfast, and a pot of tea. I would boil water in a saucepan, because I found it easier to grip the handle for pouring. Then I washed up those few things, before starting to prepare some vegetables. Everything to me was so slow and laborious that soon it was coffee time. I fought on through the preparations to dinner, and it was washing-up time again. And getting used to my new chair hampered most of these activities, anyway.

There were numerous interruptions for visits to the assessment room. Perhaps my arm supports needed re-aligning. Or a group of students wanted to talk to us. Back in the flat again, I would manfully tackle hanging out some garments on a clothes-horse outside. Dragging a bowl of wet linen on to my lap was heavy work, and my arms got tired.

At the end of a day, I was completely worn out. I lay beside Jack, aching from the day's activities. We discussed the future tentatively. Could I carry on, or would the pace prove too much? Jack had known all along that he was already contributing as much as he possibly could. But he was always a great comfort to me. "Well, don't worry, dear. If it all fails, at least we have tried, eh?"

He was playing his part well, and two small tables were

spread with his pens, paper and jewellery pieces. "I'll drop Miss Barnes a line today," he would say "Or shall I write a shopping list?"

He was ever aware of what was needed, and I appreciated his advice and encouragement. Up to my elbows in soap suds, I would call out my requirements for the week's housekeeping, budgeting with the allowance allocated us for that purpose. Little did we realise that we were setting a domestic pattern that still largely obtains for us today.

We hardly saw anyone between our allotted times of assistance. It was all part of the policy of "Planned Negligence", we came to learn. Alarm bells were everywhere, in case of difficulty, but it was against our principles to use those.

One day, Doctor Anne asked Jack how much liquid he took, and exclaimed in horror when he replied, "About four or five cups a day."

"No wonder we can't get this urinary bug out of your system. Hasn't anyone ever told you to drink plenty?"

Jack had, of course, received that advice, but pointed out that he needed help with frequent visits to the toilet.

"Can't Margaret help you with the bottle?" asked the doctor.

But this was one problem which had so far been overlooked.

"I wish I could. But the male urinals don't have a handle that I can grip," I said.

The doctor stood up, and looked thoughtful. "I'll see what we can do about that."

Next morning she returned, triumphantly holding a polythene receptacle complete with extended neck and a large curved handle. It looked ideal for the purpose. And, of course, it was. It meant another giant step towards our sought-after independence. But I could not be sure whether Jack was pleased with this latest development or not.

"Right," said Doctor Anne later, in her brisk manner. "I want you, Jack, to drink six pints of fluid a day. And you can keep an input and output record for me."

"Operation Irrigation" brought lots of practice for our new bathroom requisite. Jack was constantly concerned for me in the extra work it entailed, but my reward was to see him looking and feeling much fitter. It was a proud time for me.

In fact, my achievements were manifold. It was marvellous having so many new doors opened. The strain in my muscles was easing, and I began to cope better. I had not been used to such physical exertion, equal to someone taking up a new sporting activity. The endurance of that month's work must surely have merited a Duke of Edinburgh Award at least! But I was now learning when to rest, before real fatigue set in. And my confidence grew. There was now a distinct possibility that I would be able to manage in our own home, I was sure.

However, optimism was slightly marred towards the end of our stay, when Jack slipped into one of his despairing moods. I had encountered them before, but was still not sure how to cope with them. He just hated everything! He mooched around, and spoke only when necessary.

"Why don't you go for a ride round? I'm OK here," I said.

"I can't go on pleasure trips, while you work," he grunted.

I reassured him. "Go on. Don't be silly—I'm enjoying myself."

"Well, I'm not," he finished emphatically.

To everybody else, Jack was just "quiet", and not full of his usual jokes. We had made the acquaintance several other patients, so I suggested again that he go and talk to them.

"Get away from the domestic scene," I prompted.

He grunted again, "YOU can't get away from it."

I realised that he could not be jollied out of these moods, and preferred to be left alone.

"I can't help my moods, you know," he once apologised "It's like a black cloud comes over me—and I could kick things."

I still felt that something must be niggling Jack, and in bed that night I began to question him. He resented the interrogation. But eventually, I realised that this particular mood stemmed from feelings of utter uselessness. "Can't you see?" he pleaded, "I'm not going to be able to contribute ANYTHING to running our own home."

How well I understood his frustrations. It seemed that I was having success after success, and that Jack was accomplishing nothing. Yet while I had not married him for his usefulness around the house, he was my whole purpose for going through with this experiment at all.

I tried to comfort him once more. "I don't mind if you can't do anything. I want to be with you."

But I knew that I was not really succeeding. Obviously, Jack saw things differently. He could visualise me struggling day after day just to keep us alive, while he looked on helplessly. To the onlooker, many tasks appeared to be hard work for me, although I myself felt completely in control. I had never fooled myself that it was all going to be easy. But Jack had a habit of underestimating himself, and nothing could convince him otherwise. We decided to sleep on it.

Next morning, and with Jack still in mind, my visit to the assessment room presented an ideal opportunity to browse around the equipment on display. Sewing machines, reading aids, gadgets to help disabled people to use the telephone—all held my deep interest. Then I noticed an electric typewriter! By its side was a short stick with a rubber tip, and a flat piece at the other end. Immediately, my mind started working. If Jack held a similar stick in both hands, I was sure that he could type. This electric typewriter had an automatic carriage return, and needed a very light touch on the keys.

My thought were temporarily forestalled then, as the occupational therapist returned, saying: "Reports will be sent to your doctors, and to the Norwich Welfare Department, so how do you feel about the way you've managed here?"

I said that I had been more than satisfied.

"But do YOU think we'll be OK?", I queried.

She confirmed that modifications to a ground-floor flat would obviously be necessary, including wide doorways, lowered work surfaces and manageable cooking facilities. We would also need a hoist, and helpers to come in at peak times. This could be arranged by the various authorities in due course. We were told that our efforts at organising ourselves into a routine had been very successful.

"Now are there any other problems you can think of?"

I hesitated for a moment, remembering my idea of the typewriter.

"I wondered if you could persuade Jack to try typing?" I explained briefly what had transpired, and that Jack was feeling very inadequate. He badly needed to succeed at something just then, but almost had to be bullied into it. "He'll probably protest", I told her, "and he won't want anyone to watch him at first—neither would I, really!"

"Say no more—I get the picture," she said understandingly.

Back in the flat, I cautiously mentioned the idea to Jack. His first reaction caused me to busy myself in preparing some vegetables.

After lunch, the occupational therapist summoned Jack, and, used to unexpected calls, he complied obediently. Behind his back she winked at me knowingly. I proceeded with my tasks, concentrating hard and hoping.

At 3 p.m. I was still engrossed in my work, and listening to the radio. Jack had been gone for over an hour. When he did appear he could not conceal his pleasure, any more than he could hide the typed sheet of paper on his lap.

"Got your own way then, didn't you?" he grinned.

"Can I see what you've written?" I asked eagerly.

Expecting to see a copy of some boring piece of script, I was surprised to read a full-length letter to his mother. "Never could bear to waste your efforts, could you?" I jibed.

But I got a greater sense of achievement from this than I had from my own successes. The letter explained my "conspiracy" to get him typing, but that he was pleased to have an understanding wife who would bully him when necessary. He was full of praises for the work of the Assessment Centre as a whole.

Jack was given contacts for obtaining a reconditioned electric typewriter at the special price of £25 to disabled people. He enjoyed writing, and started wondering how to put his new-found skill to good use. His depression had lifted, and we left the Centre buoyant with success.

18: A Secret Revealed

The emptiness that followed this separation was understandably accentuated. We had enjoyed living and struggling together, and the bonds between us were thereby strengthened. But now we could only pass the waiting months away, with bright memories of our stay at the Centre, and a smile at the dilemmas we faced there.

We recalled, for instance, the day I dropped some freshly-washed liver! Trying to retrieve the wobbly substance grew more and more tiring, until Jack had to go for help.

There was also the time when the flexible tap hose was forcibly removed by a sudden surge in the water pressure. The entire kitchen floor was soaked, and my chair was skidding everywhere before I found something to knock off the tap, which I could not otherwise reach. Soon after the mopping up operation, Doctor Anne entered just in time to see a nice, clean floor.

"My word! Did you wash that floor yourself?" she exclaimed

"Well, in a way!" I said, afterwards admitting the truth.

I can laugh now, just as she did then, but it was devastating at the time.

I remembered the good times as well, like making my first curry, and hearing Jack's compliments. And I would boil an egg just firm enough to slice on to a round of bread, because I learned that Jack could not spoon it out out of its shell. I delighted in making everything to his liking.

Then there were the cosy evenings, when we would sit together by the radio. So many memories crowded our minds. Now our burning desire was for all of them to become reality.

But it remained for us to keep a simple faith in Miss Barnes and her department.

Shortly afterwards, Miss Barnes arranged another meeting, when we heard the reports from the Assessment Centre. She looked pleased and relaxed. "You've both had a successful time, according to this."

Indeed, it was reassuring to have it in writing, but could the recommendations contained in the reports be implemented? The next question was obvious, but it took time to put into words. At last, I said: "Will we be able to have a flat, then?"

Miss Barnes nodded. "Yes. But we can't say when an application can be made. And is there anywhere in Norwich you DON'T wish to live?"

We would, of course, be satisfied to live anywhere—so long as it was together. And once a flat had been allocated, Miss Barnes promised to introduce us to two young architects who would be responsible for the alterations.

The project was no longer a secret. Nothing was definite, and many questions remained unanswered. But we ventured to inform our parents and a few friends. Like us, they could scarcely believe the news.

Our most exciting meeting took place only three months later—in December 1968. Expecting to meet the architects merely to discuss necessary conversions, we were surprised to see the building plans unrolled on the table. A block of four flats was destined to be built a short distance from the hostel, and a two-bedroomed one on the ground floor had been earmarked for us. Now the plans, outlining the proposed modifications, were spread before our disbelieving eyes.

There was one big snag. Cautiously, Miss Barnes said, "But you realise that it could be a year or more before the flat is ready."

It seemed ages away. She further explained that we could choose a conversion in an existing building, but that this would certainly not be so convenient for our use. The choice was ours.

We decided to wait, and everyone breathed an almost audible sigh of relief. Several factors swayed the decision; we would be near to the city centre, have the hospital across the road, a nearby theatre, and parks. We would also be on the fringe of a Sheltered Housing Scheme. In fact, our new home would be ideally situated.

Afterwards, Jack and I discussed it all at great length. We knew the proposed building site very well. But even if building commenced immediately, which was most unlikely, a year was an awfully long time to wait. How we used that time would be all-important. One thing was certain—we had a better chance to save some money, so that we could confidently plan our bottom drawer.

To ease the long wait, Miss Barnes now arranged for a colleague, Roland, to take me to see Jack every Wednesday, thus giving us two whole days together each week.

We settled down to collecting things for our home, and Jack was allowed to store them in two large tea-chests at the hostel. Our best means of shopping was still by mail-order, and we soon had a wide assortment of household items to our credit. The project was becoming exciting in many ways, but we also got depressed sometimes—it was inevitable.

At home, whenever the subject arose, I felt awful to see Mum's uneasiness at the prospect of me leaving. We had naturally become very close, and I understood all her ups and downs, so it was going to be quite a wrench for her when I left home. She would miss our heart-to-heart talks, and the familiar sight of me sitting in bed surrounded by activity.

In his turn, Dad would find it strange not to include me in his usual daily routines. And as for Gerard—he got very upset if I simply went on holiday. So in preparing Gerard for the eventual break, I would try and make it interesting by showing him the building plans. He could also forget his sadness as he helped to wash my hair, or as he sat astride me in helping Dad to lace up my surgical support. I always answered his questions about my disability, and he soon became oblivious of my physical differences. Though slightly younger, Eileen and Joey were also curious, of course, but Gerard would soon put them right. It often amused me to hear him tell them knowledgeably "It's because she's got weak muscles, that's why." Then they would all go on chatting away merrily about everything under the sun!

Without doubt, I was going to miss them all very much.

19: Moving In

Building work on our flat commenced in February 1969. Every Wednesday, Roland drove me past the site on our way to the hostel, and I was able to report any stages of progress to Jack. Our own flat was rising slowly out of the ground. Our confidence soared even higher!

When the weather was good, Jack and I sometimes left the hostel in our powered chairs, to view the site together. We would take a camera expectantly, perhaps to find that only five more layers of bricks had been laid. One day a workman posed on his scaffolding for a photograph, when we thought that perhaps an action picture might have been more acceptable.

By late summer the roof was complete, and we feasted our eyes on the building, trying to imagine ourselves living there. But it would be some time yet.

All this time meetings had continued with Miss Barnes, the architects and ourselves. At one such meeting we were told that our hoist had been installed and that a refrigerator, spin-dryer, hob unit and a small toaster-oven made up the kitchen equipment. A special tough carpeting would be stuck to the floor in the sitting-room and in the bedroom, while vinyl tiles completed the floor-covering. As a rare privilege, we were being allowed to choose our own colour scheme.

We learned that the basic equipment and extra cost of conversion would amount to £800, most of which would probably be paid by a local charity. But for now, the Welfare Department had underwritten the full cost. It seemed an absolute fortune to us, and much as we would like to have paid, it was far beyond our means. We were more than happy to contribute in as many other ways as possible.

Another meeting decided that we should benefit from a refresher course at the Assessment Centre, and in November 1969 we were undergoing a two-weeks "dress rehearsal", as Jack called it. This time, with no pressures, we enjoyed it more.

While there, we received a letter from Miss Barnes in which she jubilantly declared: "Today, I collected the keys to the flat on your behalf, and the Department has paid some advance rent, until you are ready to move in. Meantime, we have to sort out the recruiting of your helpers. . . ."

The subject of helpers had not until this stage been confronted. Now, everything depended on finding the right people. We were given a few weeks' grace, during which the Centre decreed that I should be admitted to the hostel with Jack, in order to keep me mobile and my daily routines regular.

And so it happened. We left the Centre with everybody's good wishes ringing in our ears.

Mum had not fully come to terms with the change yet. Although she carried on as usual, she was obviously not happy and I understood her so well that it hurt me, too. Dad had in the past made no secret of his opinion: "Of course, Margaret's always been over-ambitious, you know."

His silence now was no less eloquent. I wanted to convince both them and myself that since they could not look after me forever, it was better I left home now. But my reasoning was left unspoken. Unfortunately, our family mostly coped with unhappy situations by pretending that they didn't exist. So I left home still in a state of uneasiness.

When Trevor picked me up that Friday evening, Mum had conveniently arranged to be out to avoid facing the final break. Dad seemed not to notice my departure at all. But I understood his way of coping, too. By now, Gerard had got used to the idea, and all the children shouted their cheerful goodbyes: "We'll come and see you, Margy!"

Sitting in the car, I felt cold and empty. I could have been excited. I might easily have been sad. But instead, I felt nothing.

Until finally alone with Jack, I could be myself and tears inevitably came. I poured out my feelings of guilt at leaving them all, and how terribly I would miss them. Jack was as understanding as ever. Holding my hand, he looked thoughtfully at me. "I ought to be truly proud that you care enough about me to relinquish so much."

On Jack's advice, I wrote to my parents expressing all those unspoken thoughts and feelings about leaving home. I thanked them for showing me so much care over the years. Once the letter was posted, I did feel a good deal easier.

Settling into the hostel's routine was easy enough. I knew the place, the Staff and the Residents very well, through my visits to Jack over those past nine years. A few rumours also reached our ears. "Give it a couple of months—they'll soon be back," was one.

We could only shrug in resignation at such opinions, for we ourselves could hardly be expected to make predictions. I often reflected on our physical vulnerability, realising that even a common cold could become a trial, and it was now winter time. I could not help feeling scared for the future, sometimes, as I lay quietly in my alien bed. Yet that indefinable something was urging us on—and I knew we wanted to go!

During my three weeks at the hostel, my most frequent visitors were Mum and Gerard, and gradually they helped to unpack our belongings and take them over to the flat. Larger items had already been transported by Alec, or delivered directly from the furniture stores. We spent some exciting times getting the flat ready for occupation. With the central heating already switched on, there was a warm welcome whenever we decided to travel across in our wheelchairs. Mum would dust around, put some of our clothes away and generally make the place look nice. We would eat fish and chips at our own dining table, using our own crockery, imagining we had always been there. The inevitable question was constantly being posed: "When will you move in, then?"

If only we knew! But the stock answer was simply: "As soon as we can find enough helpers."

Perhaps this was the worst time. Advertisements were entered in the local Press. Miss Barnes was interviewing a few applicants herself, before arranging for them to meet us. But very few were forthcoming, and we were feeling desperate.

"Having come this far, surely it isn't all going to fail now?" Miss Barnes was supposed to have said. Nevertheless, she always remained calmly confident to us! Then she asked if we minded having an article published on the Women's Page of the local newspaper. We were ready to agree to anything, and a full-length feature appeared, entitled "Just a little help needed."

Several more people came forward. Soon, it was agreed that an elderly couple could help us on five mornings a week, another woman settled for two mornings, whilst a friend of mine and faithful old Trevor shared the nights. The Lady Warden of the nearby Sheltered Housing Scheme was to help out with the mid-day visits and fill in at odd times, at least temporarily, until her full quota of residents had been reached.

It seemed a shaky beginning, but we now felt a strong urge to be in the flat by Christmas. The place still smelled of fresh paint and looked unlived-in, and we desperately wanted to rectify that as soon as possible. We wanted nothing more than to get on with this new life for which we had now waited two-and-a-half years, so the moment had come for naming the moving-in date.

I felt that Jack should make that choice. After all he had just staved off a serious attack of 'flu, and still had a nasty cough. Almost in defiance of this, he nominated Thursday, December 18th, 1969.

Thus after tea that day the hostel's Superintendent made a short farewell speech and we left, escorted by Alec and Trevor. We were greeted indoors by an unexpected home-coming celebration, but somehow the impact was lost in our bewilderment, and all we could do was be gracious.

Freda and Trevor stayed with us for two days and nights, to help us get acclimatised. After that, it was up to us.

20: Setting the Pace

Our first night alone might well have proved a daunting experience, but we thought little of it. With the telephone within my reach, and the alarm bell connecting us with the Lady Warden for real emergencies only, what could be safer? Our helpers had all been given keys to our front door as well. Even so, I could not resist the bewildering declaration: "Jack, I'm worried because, well, there's nothing to worry about"!

Meanwhile, our joint pension book and our rent card safely tucked away in the bureau held a special significance. Although most of our income was accounted for on the Time Sheets which Jack kept neatly for our helpers, we felt quite rich as the Lady Warden collected our money at the Post Office that first Monday!

Jack had done his homework on our budget, giving me the housekeeping to look after while he attended to other bills and calculated future expenses. It worked out most satisfactorily, and neither of us wanted more. Jack was enjoying his new role.

Christmas was fast approaching—our very first Christmas together. We had cards to send and presents to wrap, as well as some sort of life-style to organise. The days were never long enough by far. As if all this was not enough, the Spirit of Christmas appeared to us in a most unexpected way. A member of the Round Table Group arrived with a television set—something we had never dreamed of having at that time. Yet, as he placed it on our spare trolley, he even apologised for the absence of the BBC-2 channel! We were amazed and delighted simultaneously, and thanked him as well as we knew how. His wife, who accompanied him, added more goodwill by bringing some vegetables, already prepared, for our festive lunch. And there was still more to come!

On Christmas Day, just as I was about to serve our meal of chicken pieces and vegetables, the same gentleman returned with a bottle of champagne! In minutes he had completed the serving for me, and we all drank a toast to the great occasion.

We can better appreciate now the kindness shown us then. Everything was too new and strange to grasp the full meaning of it all. It was the beginning of a completely new way of life, and we could not be at all sure how it would work out.

As early as Boxing Day, our confidence was to take a hard knock. Our newly appointed morning woman failed to turn up. Waking suddenly from a deep sleep, I nudged Jack. "We've been let down. It's nine o'clock," I told him.

"Oh dear," he grunted, "I suppose we'd better ring the warden."

I managed to drag the trim-phone on to the bed, and make the call. No answer. This was most unusual. Not sure what to do next, I elected to telephone Alec, to prevent him from coming as arranged to take us to Jack's mother for the day. What a good thing Jack can memorise most of the telephone numbers we use regularly!

Before long, Alec and Laura were letting themselves in at the front door.

"Come on. We'll get you up," they announced confidently.

We were ready to accept any solution by then, and began our instructions. Pausing at one point, Alec grinned thoughtfully. "Known you for twenty years, Jack, but I've never done this before!"

Thus, we were enabled to keep to our plans. But had we known it, the Lady Warden was only walking her dogs, and would have returned in time anyway.

Miss Barnes knew nothing of this dilemma, and we decided that she deserved to be left uninterrupted over the holiday. We later discovered that our morning helper had changed her mind about the job, notifying the Welfare Department by post. The office of course was closed, so the message failed to reach us.

There was no going back now, however, and Miss Barnes herself was dressing us the following weekend.

"I hope you'll trust me to do it," she pleaded.

We were only cautious about being too much for her to handle. But she was overjoyed, and clapped her hands, when we agreed. "Come on. Where do I start, then?"

Thereby we learned another side of this wonderful person. We could not recall ever being treated with such care and respect. One would think WE were doing HER the favour!

We were to call on her services many times, until somehow we got the help we needed. Even so, she would volunteer to put us to bed extra late on the nights we wanted to attend the theatre, or go out for a meal. She was also concerned, when she called unexpectedly, if she found me trying to push the carpet-sweeper round, or struggling with the ironing. A Home Help was visiting us, but only for two hours each week, which was hardly sufficient time for our needs.

So Miss Barnes formed a habit of calling in. "I've a few minutes to spare—anything I can do?" she would ask. "I'd love to play in your kitchen!"

I was almost afraid of accepting too much help then, in case this was admitting defeat. But I was glad to allow her to dry a few dishes, and do other little jobs occasionally.

Without doubt, it was a tough time. Establishing any new routine is difficult for me, and I always seemed to be fighting the clock. After breakfast, Jack would disappear into his room to type, while I washed up. Then, when I had put some washing in to soak, as I did every day, the soap-powder would do its biological best while I assembled the necessary things to make dinner. It helped tremendously, of course, when on three days each week I could just warm up our Meals on Wheels containers. Soon it was coffee time, and so on. It may have seemed simple and straightforward to most people, but to me it was a long and tiring morning's work.

"If only I wasn't stubborn about wanting to use fresh foods.

My life would be much easier if I used frozen meals and tinned veg all the time!," I sighed.

Jack smiles at my tussles of conscience on the subject to this day.

Despite the harassing times there were some rewarding moments too. Our basic happiness was an all-important stabilising factor during this trial-and-error period.

We loved our cosy evenings together, when we could close our curtains against the outside world. Those two precious hours more than justified my long, wearying day.

To be truthful, I was my own worst enemy in those early days, when it came to being fiercely independent. It took a most insistent person to make me accept help over and above what I considered to be my quota. Family and friends were the last people I would ask, and it must have puzzled them to see me obviously needing assistance, yet determined to manage alone. Jack worried as well, constantly trying to think up ways of easing the pressures on me. It was helpful, therefore, when he managed to budget carefully enough to pay one of our women to take our washing home. This was more help than I admitted, in fact, and by keeping my culinary experiments modest, we pulled through.

By March of that first year, the elderly couple were forced to give up through illness. We were sorry to lose them, for they had formed the important basis of our original staff. Other changes meant that Trevor was doing extra duties for us, and his sister, Thelma, was also happily helping out.

Then we added another helper to our severely depleted forces. Living just around the corner with her retired husband, 64-years-old Mrs. Newby seemed the ideal person to fill our mid-day vacancy.

Though childless herself, she was motherly to us from the start. She greatly surprised herself in mastering the job, aided only by my simple instructions. Mrs. Newby soon came to understand us both very well, and her acute awareness of our needs allowed us to do our bit as well. It was often a blessing that she knew just when to take over, saying, "It's all right. I'll just do that for you."

Then quickly washing up the dinner things, she would perhaps save me an hour's work.

Nevertheless, domesticity had to be my main occupation—there was little time for anything else. One diversion, however, was talking to students about the background to our new life, and showing them what could be achieved for disabled people, given the necessary support. In fact, we were only too pleased to spread the word in this way. Thereafter, at fairly regular intervals, our small flat would be crammed with students on various courses—midwives, home helps, or maybe young people taking social studies. It was interesting for us, and we were assured that our contributions were useful.

We lost count of the number of people passing through our home during that first year. Discounting the groups of students, it was something like two hundred!

We managed to take a holiday, when Mildred and Bill had us both at their Co. Durham home for two weeks. But in spite of that break, we were living at a high pitch, though unaware of it at the time. I had been a migraine sufferer for some years, and these attacks were gradually increasing. Mercifully, they did not render me inactive for more than two hours at a time, and no drugs were needed. I just accepted it.

But I was brought to a sudden standstill in November by a severe chest infection. It was the one thing that I most dreaded, remembering my desperate battle with pneumonia all those years previously. Only then did it occur to me that I had been overdoing things, and was now being forced to ease up.

With the aid of antibiotics, my body went about its business of fighting the bug. What little strength I had to cough was helped by sitting up, so I got up in my chair as usual. I felt thoroughly miserable. But at least I was able to relax dozily, while Jack organised things around me with Mrs Newby paying extra visits to help. Also alerted to the situation, the Lady

Warden, Mrs Reeves, was required to come in during some nights, to help clear my lungs.

Triumphantly, I recovered within three weeks.

Christmas 1970 came and went, during which time we visited my family. It was the first opportunity for me to go back. It was strange to see the room rearranged where my bed had been, and to hear the familiar sounds, of the children chattering. Many memories came flooding back, but I had no regrets. In fact, this visit made me realise that I was still very much a part of the family. I welcomed that new unity. Gerard had already been calling to see us during his school lunchtimes, and Eileen paid fairly frequent visits, though she was struggling with her turbulent teens.

So we moved into our second year. Now there seemed less pressure upon us to do well. It had been vitally important to us to "make it" in that first twelve months. We were always setting the pace—always gauging our own efforts against what we thought might be expected of us. In this demanding situation, any accomplishment brought satisfaction. Then, having achieved our aims this far, we became more confident. Even the failure of my powered chair was not the desperate disaster I once feared. Slowly, our daily activities increased. Our talks to the students continued, and I began to do some jewellery repairs. We bought a daily newspaper, and actually found time to read it. Realising that I enjoyed making my own clothes, Jack managed to buy a secondhand electric sewing machine. Then we both became active committee members of the St Raphael Club.

All the time, Miss Barnes was in regular contact, though keeping unobtrusively in the background.

21: Jack Falls Ill

Then Jack developed a severe pain in his right side. I remember it all so vividly. It was a Wednesday evening in June, and we had just returned from the Club. Jack looked awful, and was glad to get to bed, thinking he might feel better after the night's rest.

Indeed, the next day Jack said that he felt fine again, and got on with some more jewellery pieces in his workroom. However, bending over his bench put a strain on his side and by midday the pain had returned. It got worse quite quickly, and he actually asked to go back to bed. This most unusual request underlined the severity of his discomfort.

I contacted the doctor, and he arrived within half an hour. Judging by Jack's condition, and testing the urine sample which we had the presence of mind to keep, the G.P. thought there might be a stone in the kidney. Pethadin was administered, and Jack was temporarily out of his misery. I was relieved to see him lying there all serene, his face free of that terrible pain. Helpless to do anything physically, I could but watch and wait. Mrs Reeves was available if needed, but it was profoundly frustrating not being able to help Jack myself. I sat by the bed, completely resigned to what was happening. Jack, usually so alive and in control, was now out to the world—and to me.

I wondered if this was how it would all finish. Was this indeed the beginning of the end of our new life together? Not that I thought Jack was going to die—but what if this illness should be a long one? I could not nurse him. When he lay in bed, I could not even reach out and touch him. And the doctor had hinted at surgery. How long would it take for Jack to get over that, and would he ever be fit again? All these questions went round and round in my head, as I continued my watch.

Meanwhile, Jack was still snoring away, though not in a normal kind of sleep. His face was grey, and twitched now and then. Sometimes his eyes opened blankly. I did wonder if he really was asleep, or semi-consciously aware of everything. So I talked calmly at intervals about everyday things.

"I'll just draw the curtains."

"Please say if you want me to get help."

"Just going in the other room, Jack. Back in a minute."

I even switched on the radio cricket commentary—anything to maintain a relaxed atmosphere. I tried not to dwell on the black side, pushing the morbid thoughts to the back of my mind.

But when the doctor returned at 7p.m., his quiet but meaningful enquiry reiterated all my fears.

"Now, what d'you say, Jack? Would you like a bed in hospital overnight?"

Jack, still only half awake, admitted to having the pain. The silence while he considered the question seemed to last far too long. The old conviction that disabled people were denied the right to control their own lives came storming back to me. To my surprise, Jack's reply came firm and clear : "No, thanks. I'll be all right."

I waited—convinced that the doctor would insist we were in no position to cope under these circumstances. Instead, he patted Jack on the shoulder, saying, "All right, you know best. But I'll give you another injection for the pain, and call back in the morning."

I breathed a little sigh of relief. I was pleased that Jack obviously felt secure enough to stay here at home. It was also reassuring to know that the doctor trusted us. My optimism was returning. I suddenly knew that we could win this fight together, as we had so many others.

By now I had become very cool-headed. Once in his drugged state, Jack was no longer able to issue instructions for making him comfortable. How glad I was that we knew each other's needs so well. As it was, Jack would not have complained at all, but I realised that his limbs should not be allowed to go numb. Mrs. Reeves' nursing training confirmed this, and she volunteered to give Jack a wash.

"He should feel easier after that, I think," she said, caringly. "And he must keep drinking, you know, my dear," she added.

Rising to the command, I said, "Perhaps a cup of tea would be a change from the fruit squash?" Waiting for the kettle to boil, I then realised that I was in need of some refreshment myself, having had nothing since lunch. I prepared myself a sandwich. It would not do to neglect my own needs at a time like this.

Eventually, Mrs Reeves got him into what I considered to be a comfortable sitting position, supported all round with pillows. But in any case, he was now snoring contentedly.

Miss Barnes came in that evening, and insisted on staying for as long as it took to settle us both down for the night. Jack's drug was wearing off, and to our astonishment, he suddenly said, in an alert tone, "Right. I think I'll lie down now, please."

Miss Barnes convulsed with laughter, grateful for the excuse to release some of the tremendous build-up of tension.

He talked more cheerfully saying that the pain had now subsided. He accepted another drink, and was soon snuggled down on his favourite right side.

It was well past midnight before Miss Barnes left, and I promised to telephone her with any news. We managed to fall asleep and, miraculously, the night passed without incident.

Next morning, Jack insisted on getting up. The pain was not too bad, and only half a tablet of pethadin sufficed to keep it at bay. The doctor paid an early visit, and seemed pleased with Jack's obvious improvement. Thankfully, surgery was considered unnecessary but Jack was given an appointment at the hospital to make sure.

Though frightening at the time, that short, sharp episode served to remind us of yet another achievement. The hospital examination later showed no stones in the kidney, and there has been no recurrence of the pain. But Jack has faithfully followed the doctor's advice to keep up a large liquid intake daily.

Overcoming this nasty experience boosted our confidence. We had coped with a fairly serious degree of illness, without relinquishing our independence. The least we could do was to care for our wellbeing as well as we knew how, and by reading, and checking with the doctor, we set the pattern for our present state of good health. I never become over-complacent, realising full well that we are but frail human beings, after all. But while the feeling of wellbeing exists for us both, I thank goodness itself, and enjoy life.

Soon after Jack's bout of kidney trouble, we both accepted Mildred and Bill's second invitation to holiday with them—this time, in London. In anticipation of this, Roland offered to redecorate our lving-room, and brought wallpaper books and paint charts for our perusal. We spent a very pleasant time choosing the varying shades of green which we like so much, and in our absence, Roland and his wife set to work. When we got back, we barely recognised the place looking so clean and different. It was a lovely welcome.

22: We Lose a Dear Friend

The Second Anniversary of our move into the flat was near at hand. It certainly deserved a celebration of some kind, and we even considered throwing a big party. But eventually, we settled for a quiet drink with Miss Barnes. Of all those involved, we knew that she shared our feelings of achievement more deeply than most.

We had not succeeded by ourselves, that was certain, and Miss Barnes still represented a reliable force behind us. Whenever anything cropped up, she was but a telephone call away. When a replacement was needed amongst our helpers, she was the one to advertise, and to select a suitable few for us to interview.

Our dependence on Miss Barnes was not obvious, however, and her holidays presented no problems to us. Nevertheless, it did not alter the fact that we began to relax a little more when she was working, and readily available. Calling in at least once a week for a chat, she continued to help out on our required late nights. She always made a gentle entry, bowing her unusually tall frame almost reverently as she did so.

I had noticed that Miss Barnes seemed unwell. Jack thought that perhaps she was working too hard. We mentioned this during our evening's celebration, when her pallor and pained expression seemed more apparent. She admitted to having rather severe abdominal pains, saying, "Hiatus hernia, the doctor said."

We expressed our genuine concern.

Later on, as we lay in bed, Jack and I mulled over the evening again, continually reminded that something was definitely wrong with Miss Barnes. Instinctively, thereafter, we began easing up on her. We had been relying on her to a large extent, but now our only concern was for herself. Our own feelings of insecurity were forgotten. Naturally, she always put on a brave face, going about her duties in characteristic style.

Two weeks later, Miss Barnes remained casual when informing us that she was to visit a specialist. "I think I have an ulcer."

I was equally cheerful in my approach—but even then, I had feelings of foreboding.

She was so aware of our need for her that her worry would be more for us than herself. In fact she insisted on putting us to bed one more time, before being admitted into hospital for an exploratory operation in January 1972.

"Can we come and see you—we can easily get across the road?"

Her face lit up immediately. "Oh, yes. You must."

Thus, we visited her on the following Saturday. Gerard, who had to see us safely into the hospital, stood awkwardly as any sixteen-year-old lad would, while we chatted away. Miss Barnes looked out of place in that old hospital day-room, so much like those which Jack recalled. We saw how thin she had become, sitting wrapped in a dressing-gown, and nursing our posy of violets on her lap. It was difficult not to betray our feelings of deep sadness as we left, and only managing to say: "We'll be thinking about you."

We went to see her again the day after the operation.

"Probably only removed my appendix," she said, brightly.

More seriously, the truth was known. She told us that there was a malignant growth on the pancreas, which would be treated with radium.

We visited Miss Barnes frequently, always taking Spring flowers which she loved. Sometimes, we found her making a brave effort and sitting on top of the bed, or in an armchair. But her skin was parched and yellow, and her eyes shone too brightly. At first, she would converse interestedly, and when everything else failed, she knew that Jack could easily be stirred into airing his views on the state of Norwich City's football team!

Then her expression changed, as that awful feeling of nausea returned. It was a pitiful sight. Then, talking did not come easy to any of us. She would hold my hand quietly, as we tried to find everyday things to say.

Her courage amazed us. Never a single word of protest passed her lips, even though she realised her fate. She maintained her appearance as far as she was able, once saying: "But I'm so very thin, my dear. Do I look as dreadful?" I shook my head, and smiled my reassurance. "You do look very ill. But even illness doesn't mask a person's character. You have an air of peace about you. And your eyes look alive." She smiled at my words, then closed her eyes to rest. What I had said was all true. Indeed, despite her condition, her gentle, caring nature showed through.

Then one morning Miss Barnes telephoned from the hospital. Her speech was slurred and broken, as she explained that she was going into a Hospice in London.

Maintaining her usual optimism, she said: "People do come out of there sometimes, you know."

There was a short pause, before she made her gentle conclusion. "Bye, bye. Bless you both."

Those were the very last words we heard her say.

I felt that I just had to write to her at once, setting her mind at rest about us. We reassured her that she had shown us how to live. Realising that Miss Barnes was instrumental in getting us established, we wanted her to know that she had not let us down, nor left a job unfinished. We hoped that she would not regret becoming involved with us, even though it was, to a large extent, beyond her call of duty. I told her that we always admired her ideals, and recognised her deep respect for human dignity in the individual. We would endeavour to live by those ideals.

Subsequently, a telephoned message from her closest friend

told us, "Elizabeth says, 'Tell Margaret and Jack their letter was perfect. They said all the right things'."

Miss Barnes died a week later—at Easter. Though we more or less accepted the inevitable, it was still a terrible blow. We had lost our mainstay, and a true friend. My final expression of respect was to read a Lesson at her Memorial Service. Miss Barnes was the most genuine and dedicated social worker.

23: Decisions and Reflections

With Miss Barnes' death still weighing heavily upon us, we were now faced with another important decision. Our friend Roland had offered Jack the chance to apply for a clerical post at a newly built, all-purpose centre for the disabled. It was his very first opportunity in a whole lifetime of a real job. Someone was needed to allocate rooms, deal with the office work and generally co-ordinate activities. Jack had the necessary organising ability—but did he have the physical stamina? It was an opportunity which could not be rejected lightly. We discussed it for days on end, often wishing we had Miss Barnes' sound advice to call on.

"She would know whether it was right for us," we would sigh.

But thinking along those lines was futile. In fact we realised at this point that we were suddenly thrown well and truly on to our own feet. I tried not to put pressures on him in any direction. I wanted only what he wanted. The status of earning for us both would mean a tremendous boost to Jack's self-esteem. On the other hand he pointed out that we would have to leave home each morning unusually early for us. There would be lunches to pack, and evening meals to prepare. In no time, we would be going to bed! We might also be asked to work on Saturday mornings.

Eventually Jack decided that he could not apply for the job. He needed a more flexible routine than this would allow. He also felt that I was already fully committed, domestically. Only then did I admit to having my own reservations on the matter. Within our own environment we were capable of achieving a lot. But it had to be in our time, and at our pace. So, writing a formal letter to Roland declining the offer, Jack thanked him for the privilege, at least, of turning down his first ever chance of employment!

Altogether it was a time of reflection for us both. We felt established in our way of life, but somehow something was missing—a sense of purpose perhaps? No doubt the past sixteen years had conditioned us in some way to exerting ourselves. We had been struggling against a system which refused to accept that disabled people could even have ambitions, let alone expect them to be realised!

But all this was behind us now. Whilst the loss of Miss Barnes cast a dark shadow over us, our own feelings of accomplishment could not be obliterated completely. Now we did have control over our own lives. Of course, we depended on people, and disciplined ourselves to fit in with our helpers' visits. But everyone has some sort of framework within which they must operate—their work routines, their family and social commitments. Indeed we now felt a part of the community. But we did feel the need of something more.

We discussed these thoughts and feelings frequently, usually as we lay peacefully in bed at night. First, Jack might sigh: "If only I could've been the bread-winner, maybe I'd feel different. What use am I to society?"

My thoughts would wander in another direction. "I suppose the natural progression for most couples at this stage would be to start a family?" I observed, "Nature is no fool. She even puts such instincts into the likes of me!"

Jack had always said that he would not have wanted children of his own, though he enjoyed them generally. "But I wouldn't deny you anything, of course," he told me.

But I quickly reassured him.

With such a disease as ours, I judged it morally wrong to have children of our own, quite apart from all the physical hazards of a pregnancy. I would not complicate our lives further. I was simply trying to find explanations for our sudden lack of purpose. We obviously had to look away from ourselves for that feeling of fulfilment, for lately we had been indulged to a much larger degree than we had ever expected.

Consequently, when the St Raphael Club were needing a new secretary, Jack was happy to take the position. He proved to be a conscientious secretary in his limited way, and his work led him into many interesting aspects of running a club of this kind, with its own premises and varied membership. Although voluntary work was not exactly what he had had in mind, he felt that he was making a useful contribution.

Meetings were being held at a new all-purpose Centre, run by the local authority, for disabled people from all groups to suggest suitable activities. We wanted to see something organised for children with all kinds of handicap, together with their able-bodied brothers and sisters. We ourselves had experienced enough segregation, in "special" schools, "special" clubs, and even separate societies for separate disabilities. We liked the idea of bringing all children together.

By a timely coincidence we then read in a magazine about the Toy Libraries Association, and out of curiosity sent for details. Toy libraries stock toys, and lend them out, in much the same way as another library might lend books, or records.

It seemed just what we needed here in Norwich. Before long we had contacted the Social Services Department to discover what legalities were involved, and whether running a toy library really was within our capabilities. It all seemed straightforward, so Jack and I set to work in spreading the idea and writing numerous begging letters.

In six months, helpful friends and acquaintances had joined us in forming a steering committee, and we had raised £300. We opened a bank account, and felt quite humble as cheques came flooding in, usually made payable to us in the absence of an official title for our toy library! It was all happening so quickly. We were suddenly in the news again—but this time for a different reason.

With Gerard being so closely involved with our lives, it was fitting that he should also come on to the toy library committee. He was used to taking me into the city on Saturdays to get my weekly shopping. Now, he was with me in a group of committee members out to buy toys.

The new Centre were pleased to co-operate in storing our toys, and welcomed our using their main hall for our fortnightly sessions. The Norfolk and Norwich Toy Library opened to the public on March 20th, 1973. At first, business was slow, but as news of our existence spread, children would arrive with their individual families, or in small groups from their special schools. Helpers' children also mixed in well, and some form of integration began taking place.

As often happens, we slipped innocently into this new commitment. Little did we realise what an important part of our lives the Toy Library would become. We had found our new sense of purpose!

24: Possum Means I AM ABLE

It seemed incredible that only the previous year we had been finding barely sufficient time to keep ourselves functioning. Now, our lives were so full of activity. After all our fears, it was both gratifying and relieving to know that ours would not be just a day-to-day existence. There would be time and energy for other things, and the Toy Library needed both.

There was a constant flow of letters and phone calls, in connection either with the Club or the Toy Library. Jack's typewriter worked overtime, while only I could use the telephone. Hardly a day went by without our being involved in some aspect of our secretarial partnership, and we were carried along on a wave of enthusiasm.

Then as Jack began concentrating even harder on promoting the Toy Library he had little choice but to relinquish his secretaryship in the St Raphael Club, where he had gained a valuable two years' experience. His loyalties were torn, but once satisfied that the Club was left in good hands he could get properly to grips with cementing this new project of ours.

Officially, I was the secretary of the Toy Library and Jack the treasurer but as usual, he did all the writing, as well as keeping an eye on everything else. The amount of publicity literature being produced surprised us both, and we now had the Toy Library's own posters displayed at many points in the city and surrounding districts. We worked hard, but it must be said that the rewards were great. There was much good-natured debate on what toys should or should not be purchased, selecting from local stores or from mail-order catalogues. Now, the Toy Library became the subject of most of our periodic public talks, with only an occasional request for us to speak about ourselves.

In fact our own routine had faded unobtrusively into the background, to be thrown into relief again only by the necessity to advertise for a new helper. Even this was not the startling jolt it used to be. But we did turn our attention inwards upon ourselves again before very long.

It happened as an indirect result of our need for a new helper that we met Ursula, who offered to help out while we were advertising. She soon became a friend, and we called on her services quite often after that, though not in the same way as we had with Miss Barnes, whom she had known.

As an occupational therapist with the new Social Services Department, Ursula's task was to supply necessary aids to disabled people, both young and old, in their homes. It was Ursula, therefore, who told us about some special equipment called "Possum". We had vaguely heard of this somewhat futuristic device, but did not realise that we ourselves might possibly qualify for its free issue from the Department of Health and Social Security. However, Ursula thought that we should try, and explained how to apply through our GP.

It was over a year before we had the equipment finally installed, but it proved to be well worth waiting for, and although mainly for Jack's benefit, it also helped me indirectly a great deal.

Possum Equipment is an electronic device which enables severely disabled people to control various activities in the home. A sustained sucking motion on a tube activates lights, television, radio, and releases an electric lock on the front door. But by far the greatest boon to Jack was the added ability to answer the telephone, and to dial calls. In discovering the wonders of Possum, he eventually saved up to buy himself a tape-recorder, and later obtained a page-turner for his books.

Each selection is made from an illuminated panel, pausing on the suction tube when the appropriate function is reached. If the user cannot see the panel, he counts a certain number of bleeps. The full range of facilities was available from a similar tube in our bedroom, and also from the small micro-switch situated in the living-room.

Jack was immensely pleased with this new found independence. "Now you can go out, without worrying about me," he observed, "And when you're busy in the kitchen, you can leave me to answer the door, and the phone."

I always grudged interruption to my kitchen activities. Just when I was conveniently placed at the sink, the telephone or the doorbell would call me away. And Jack had always longed to be more practically useful to me—and now he could be. I was overjoyed for both our sakes. Thus, while seated at his typewriter, Jack could be in virtual control of the whole household!

We marvelled frequently at the powers of Possum, and the more so as the Toy Library brought increased use of the telephone. As an off-shoot of this ongoing business, the Social Services Department suggested that we could perhaps co-ordinate Playschemes for mentally handicapped children during school holidays. These children could not be included in other playschemes because they needed special supervision; but their parents needed a break.

So we started by contacting local schools and colleges for helpers; we needed a one-to-one ratio of helpers to children. Then we soon became entangled in the machinery of local authority in negotiating for transport and financial grants. This was something for which we had not been prepared, and we had to learn new assertive skills.

We still derive great pleasure from these playschemes, despite the hurly-burly, and the worries involved in catering for some forty severely mentally handicapped children. I attend the sessions as they are held, during the Easter and Summer holidays, organising the girls with their daily protégés, and making sure that the play leaders have sufficient materials to work with. Meantime, Jack is left holding the home fort from before nine in the morning. He deals with the never ending paperwork, and also organises our helpers into preparing our lunch for when I return at one o'clock. These are among the few occasions when Jack and I have to do things independently of each other.

Soon after our Possum equipment had been installed, we became members of the Possum Users' Association, an organisation run by the disabled for the disabled. But it certainly did not occur to us at the time that the PUA would be the source of another invaluable amenity for us, and other disabled people in our area.

However, on August 19th, 1976, we took delivery of a smart red Ford 90 Transit dormobile, complete with automatic lift on the back, presented to us by the Possum Users' Association.

It seemed too good to be true, and we were absolutely delighted. The Press were invited to attend the presentation, and the usual publicity followed.

The PUA tax and insure the vehicle for any responsible person with a current driving licence. We have to keep it serviced and properly maintained, and to lend it out for carrying other disabled people. Two wheelchair passengers can be accommodated, which is ideal for us. Transport is always a problem with those confined to wheelchairs, and this van has certainly added a whole new dimension to our lives.

One of the many benefits of this convenient means of transport was that I could join an Adult Education Course for a couple of terms, deriving great pleasure from dabbing away at still-life oil-paintings.

Likewise, our theatre trips increased, and visits to restaurants with friends became an easier proposition.

Having had one door opened, it seemed that countless others were leading us further into the world of "normal" people. Small wonder that we often found ourselves making incredulous comparisons with our earlier years!

25: The Book

Clearly, we liked being busy, and people would sometimes comment: "You two seem to do more than some fit people I know!" We could hardly agree with them, when our slow pace could never compete with the quick movements of those around us. But to each other, we did from time to time come back to the idea that perhaps we had a story to tell. It was the prospect of laboriously writing it all down that always deterred us from making a start. I imagined that an autobiographer would need to become too inward-looking. Or on the other hand, could we be objective enough? So, once more, we were trying to make a decision, and meet a challenge.

"It would take us ages, and I wouldn't know where to begin," I'd say.

Jack, however, was a little more enthusiastic. "Can't see where we'll find the time—but I'd like to try! You just scribble something down, and I'll make it presentable," he encouraged.

Thus, with Jack tenaciously sticking to the task whenever possible, we gradually formed the basis for this book. Many a time, he had to prompt me into another effort "I've nearly finished what you've done—when can you write some more?"

I would quickly grab a pen and paper at odd moments between chores, or settle down to writing for an hour in the evenings. To begin with it was a very peace-meal effort on my part, I was so often disturbed when I dearly wanted to have a long spell at my writing. Then there were times when I picked up a sheet of Jack's beautifully typed manuscript, and erupted indignantly: "You can't put that. Oh, heck. We do sound a pious pair."

The atmosphere got very heated until we both learned to

give and take a little. After all, it had to be a joint creation, and Jack could not be expected to be a mere copy-typist.

Next, we became members of the Norwich Writers' Circle, pleased to have the sound advice and interest of both established and aspiring writers. Well meaning criticism often resulted in the destruction of several days' work! But gritting our teeth determinedly, we pressed on, having made up our minds to complete the task, and properly, come what may.

For some considerably long time, "The Book" became a standing joke. Whenever we met an acquaintance, the inevitable question arose: "How's that book coming along?"

We often welcomed the reminder, having told everybody for the secret purpose of not being able to back down, I do believe.

We puzzled our heads for a title for the book.

"Nothing corny, please!" I would insist.

But needless to say, there were many suggestions, one idea being *Love on Wheels*. I groaned! Were people just being downright rude? *All Part of Living* was a little better, but I was still not satisfied. We considered several other titles before arriving at the present one.

There were repeated and unavoidable breaks from writing, when a run of other work demanded Jack's typewriter.

"We need to lock ourselves away for a whole year to finish this book—like any other self-respecting writer would," he said impatiently.

Then gradually, as we moved through the story, with several chapters behind us we worked with renewed enthusiasm. Whenever we sipped a glass of our home-made wine, the toast was: "To The Book."

26: A Death in the Family

Just after Easter 1978, my father spent a week in hospital undergoing tests which revealed that he had cancer of the stomach and liver. It was a terrible blow to us all to realise that even an operation was futile. But Dad accepted his fate courageously, almost defiantly referring to his cancer as casually as people talk about their arthritis.

Though almost seventy years old, Dad had kept active, carrying himself in the upright fashion of his RSM training. Accompanied by Mum, he visited us every Friday doing thoughtful little favours in my kitchen, such as setting the machine going for my week's washing. He would often peel all my vegetables for the weekend, and when he did he always made the touching gesture of walking through to pop a piece of raw carrot into my mouth!

He would chat about his own wine-making, long before I was interested in taking it up myself.

Dad was gentle and understanding with Jack. At lunch time, he would cut up Jack's food, before tucking a serviette under his chin. Dad had not shown real approval of our marriage at the start, too concerned about its possible failure and the subsequent hurt for us. But seeing us established in our own flat, he obviously felt secure about the situation. He could not bring himself to say as much to our faces, but I was aware that he spoke proudly of us to others.

Dad became very weak during the last fortnight of his life, and when he was confined to bed the family watched by him constantly. During the final days I managed to visit Dad several times, when Trevor or my brothers were able to carry me upstairs to the first-floor flat. Jack came with me on one occasion. As we watched his tired, grey face, my thoughts could not help but wander back almost twenty-two years to the day when Dad had cycled to Dereham with the news of Gerard's birth. Now, Gerard was helping Mum to tend Dad's needs to the end.

Dad died on Friday, May 12th, at home, as was his wish and with the family in attendance.

Gerard aptly summed it up later, when he said: "Dad taught us how to live—and he taught us how to die."

27: A Typically Busy Day

Life, for us, just had to go on. After the natural mourning of my father's death, our daily routine went ahead at its usual hectic pace.

Tuesday is Toy Library day, and perhaps the most crowded schedule of all. Ten-thirty a.m. sees me trundling across to the Centre in my powered chair, to discover that proceedings are already well under way. Trusty helpers have prepared the room, which entails wheeling out six large cupboards stacked with toys, inflating a big air-mattress, erecting the sturdy Wendy House, and displaying bikes, trolleys and various toys of mobility. My task is then to chat to young mothers with handicapped children and/or toddlers, and listen with interest to their latest developments. Around me, the regular volunteers are entertaining the children, and keeping files on toys borrowed.

At 12 noon, the playgroup sessions ends. Some stalwarts stay on, and with the tidying up completed, we munch our packed lunches, brought for the occasion, and talk over the morning's happenings. Before long, Jack arrives with my brother Gerry, as he now prefers to be called.

The afternoon is more boisterous, as it caters for the older children from the special schools and units, with attendances of up to 40 at one time! Through the noise, Jack keeps a records book of all transactions, including the loans of specialised books and advisory leaflets, and our own publicity literature.

My role becomes more varied, as perhaps I meet a group of students from the local college; talk to one or two of the children's teachers; help to check jig-saws and games for missing pieces; advise new helpers; or simply do a stint on the filing system, alongside Gerry. Occasionally, we are called to pose for a Press photographer as a presentation is made to the Toy Library by a generous individual or organisation.

As people filter away, the great clearing-up process begins, and everyone pitches in. Jack and I can contribute very little in this respect, except to give guidance where bits and pieces belong. But by co-operation of many willing hands, the 30-foot long hall is soon looking its spick-and-span self once more.

Then Gerry loads us into the van for our short journey home.

It never ceases to amaze us that we should actually have initiated such a rewarding and worthwhile pursuit. Yet the efficiency of our helpers still allows us the occasional day off, and it is gratifying to us to know that the Toy Library will carry on functioning in our absence.

Once home, we eat our meal while watching the television news, and then settle on our own to read the papers, or work on some more writing. Usually, evenings are our least disturbed times, endeavouring as we do to cram all our commitments into the daytime, whether it be entertaining visitors; going out giving talks about ourselves or the Toy Library; or merely attending to routine correspondence. Intermingled with everything else, of course, come the more down-to-earth details of general housekeeping duties.

Many is the time I interrupt Jack's typing with a despairing remark like: "Oh, what can we have for tea?" quickly followed by, "And who was it on the phone just now?"

And with a full day behind us, bed-time comes when our night helper, Pat, arrives at about 9.30 p.m., and the routine comes almost automatically. A combination of mechanical hoist and a willing pair of hands works wonders—even hands already tired from a day's chores elsewhere. Hands carefully washing, undressing, and even obliging to a simple request, such as "Will you scratch my back, please?"

The process of settling us down is invariably accompanied

by jokes, and some discussion on the day's events. We hear about highlights in our helper's family life.

"My little girl is in the school play this week, and she's absolutely thrilled."

We talk over points in the news, and have our friendly disagreements. These are just normal interactions between normal personalities. And all the time those hands work ever so patiently, moving this leg or that arm "just a fraction", until we are nestled into positions which we know from years of experience will be comfortable all through the night.

After about an hour, Pat leaves the house.

"Goodnight. Thanks a lot, Pat. See you tomorrow," we call finally.

Jack activates his Possum, and the last light is extinguished. For a few moments perhaps, we are silent, revelling in the sheer comfort of bed after sitting all day long.

Perhaps Jack then leads a revision on plans for a forthcoming event in the Toy Library, or discusses something which needs attention on the van. Maybe I tell him about the people I met, and things we have done at my evening class in Art.

Whichever way the conversation takes us, sleep soon comes. Gone are the times when Jack lay awake half the night pondering over various things, simply because he was not tired enough to sleep! Now, we are both well and truly exhausted. But it is a healthy tiredness, which follows each satisfying day. We never look too far into the future, but take life as it comes and enjoy each day to its fullness.

"I think I'm going to sleep now. Goodnight, Love," yawns Jack.

"Goodnight, darling. Love you."

28: Simple Pleasures

As our days are full, so are our pleasures many. We never fail to find excitement in the everyday things, like observing the antics of birds clamouring round our bird-table. We enjoy sampling a new recipe, using our home-grown tomatoes tenderly raised from seeds. There is added meaning to drinking home-made wines, while spending our favourite evenings together with radio or television for company. A selection of music cassettes makes a fitting atmosphere to browsing through our stamp collection. Our interest in the live theatre has increased, and we now attend more regularly.

We even enjoyed the challenge of coping with a power workers' strike, when our total dependence on the supply of electricity for everything including our hoist and central heating presented considerable difficulties. But we had warmth from a paraffin heater, and I managed to make soups and hot drinks on a small camping stove. However, one advantage I did have over most other people. Having a 12-volt battery underneath me meant that Alec could rig me up with a bulb and flex, and my light travelled with me! Conversely, when the "lightning strikes" were on, I am sure that few other people lived in fear of being suspended in mid-air on a hoist! But our helpers and friends adjusted their times accordingly, and in fact the crisis was averted.

We take a keen interest in watching my brothers' children grow up, and perhaps most especially in Eileen's little family. We also follow Gerry's aspirations to become a Social Worker. As a single man still, his only true commitment is to his work as an Assistant Warden in a hostel for homeless young men. But twice a week he will still interrupt his own social life, to become our official night helper. Apart from this, he pops in to see us most days, anyway.

Jack regrets that those unavoidable circumstances of the past caused him to become more remote from his family than I from mine. But he is always pleased to hear news of his sisters' families, from a telephone call or an occasional visit, or when meeting his mother at the Club on Wednesdays. Jack's biggest regret is that his dear old grandparents did not live to see his achievements.

Naturally, we are still closely involved with Freda and Trevor and their children, Andrew now thirteen, and nine-year-old Rachel. We look forward to our exchange visits to their home, and to the home of Trevor's sister Thelma, her husband David, and their offspring James and Paul, who are our god-sons.

With the opportunity to share so many other people's children, it seems we were denied little after all. We have witnessed a baby's first steps; an infant's first paintings; an older child's struggle with homework. We have encountered tantrums; children's ailments; the harassed mother; the proud mother of a perfect new-born babe. And, alas, we have shared the deep sadness of a mother bereaved of a young handicapped child. In all, we have been fortunate and privileged to enter the childrens' world, without having the responsibilities of bringing them up!

In many ways, since coming to this new life, we have been greedy for experience. Perhaps we were simply wanting to make up for lost time. Yet we know that, without those lost years, today would not be so satisfying. Despite our voracious appetite for life, and all it brings, we still relish every morsel slowly and gratefully.

One often reads of disabled people as being the under-privileged, the forgotten ones, and we certainly know of some ourselves who could fall into those categories. But for us, the luck changed: public attitudes improved and society developed all at the right time. Above all, we met Elizabeth Barnes, who was willing to put her trust in our limited abilities and take a risk. And we were prepared to take a step into the unknown.

We could not possibly know what lay ahead. We had to take a chance—the chance of our lifetime. It could have failed so miserably.

"Why do you seem to attempt the impossible?" we have been asked.

Our answer is simple.

"Because we usually find it possible!"

All those years ago, when we first held hands so shyly in that old hospital room, we could never have imagined that this new world of ours was even remotely possible. Being close to each other every day of our lives was all we ever wanted.

We cannot take THAT pleasure for granted even now.